Praise for Getting Past the Affair

"A worthy and important contribution to understanding and helping couples face one of the worst problems in a relationship."
—John M. Gottman, PhD, author of *The Seven Principles for Making Marriage Work*

"The hurt lingered for what felt like forever, but our marriage was too precious to just give up on it. Working through understanding how it happened, and how to finally move past it and recover, was the most important thing. We couldn't have made it without the program in this book."
—Ann and Patrick O.

"It's easy to find simplistic, judgmental advice about dealing with affairs—but hard to find a book like this. Far and away the most important resource to help you understand the meaning of the affair and make healthy decisions about how to move on."
—Barry McCarthy, PhD, coauthor of *Rekindling Desire*

"After the revelation of the affair, we were both overwhelmed with extreme emotions. The step-by-step approach outlined in this book gave us a structured and caring means to get through the first couple of months and work to understand how we got to this low point in our marriage. We made it through a very tough time and have a stronger relationship now, due to our greater understanding of both ourselves and each other. Without question, the strategies in this book saved our marriage!"
—John and Sarah H.

"If an affair has left you feeling devastated, this book can put you on a path toward healing by providing hope, direction, and clarity. The second edition takes an already classic resource and makes it even better for couples with diverse backgrounds and types of relationships. This is *the* book that I recommend to anyone struggling with infidelity."
—Anthony L. Chambers, PhD, ABPP, former president, American Academy of Couple and Family Psychology

Getting Past the Affair

Also Available for Professionals

Clinical Handbook of Couple Therapy, Sixth Edition
Jay L. Lebow and Douglas K. Snyder, Eds.

Couple-Based Interventions
for Military and Veteran Families: A Practitioner's Guide
Douglas K. Snyder and Candace M. Monson, Eds.

Helping Couples Get Past the Affair: A Clinician's Guide
*Donald H. Baucom, Douglas K. Snyder,
and Kristina Coop Gordon*

Treating Difficult Couples: Helping Clients
with Coexisting Mental and Relationship Disorders
Douglas K. Snyder and Mark A. Whisman, Eds.

Getting Past the Affair

A Program to Help You Cope, Heal,
and Move On—Together or Apart

SECOND EDITION

Douglas K. Snyder, PhD
Kristina Coop Gordon, PhD
Donald H. Baucom, PhD

THE GUILFORD PRESS
New York   London

To all the couples who shared with us their intimate struggles of recovery from an affair. Your testimonies of trial and triumph bear witness to the healing potential of love, commitment, and hard work.

Copyright © 2023 The Guilford Press
A Division of Guilford Publications, Inc.
370 Seventh Avenue, Suite 1200, New York, NY 10001
www.guilford.com

The information in this volume is not intended as a substitute for consultation with healthcare professionals. Each individual's health concerns should be evaluated by a qualified professional.

Printed in the United States of America

Last digit is print number: 9   8   7   6   5   4   3   2   1

Library of Congress Cataloging-in-Publication Data

Names: Snyder, Douglas K., author. | Gordon, Kristina Coop, author. |
    Baucom, Donald H., author.
Title: Getting past the affair : a program to help you cope, heal, and move
    on—together or apart / Douglas K. Snyder, Kristina Coop Gordon,
    Donald H. Baucom.
Description: Second edition. | New York, NY : The Guilford Press, 2023. |
    Includes bibliographical references and index.
Identifiers: LCCN 2023020395 | ISBN 9781462547487 (paperback) |
    ISBN 9781462552832 (hardcover)
Subjects: LCSH: Marital psychotherapy. | Adultery—Psychological aspects.
Classification: LCC RC488.5 .S627 2023 | DDC 616.89/1562—dc23/eng/20230527
LC record available at *https://lccn.loc.gov/2023020395*

Contents

PART III

How Can We Move Forward?

Purchasers of this book can download and print an enlarged
version of the Worksheet for Summarizing Factors Related
to the Affair at *www.guilford.com/snyder2-forms* for personal
use or use with clients (see copyright page for details).

Authors' Notes
and Acknowledgments

This book evolved from decades of clinical practice, our own empirical research, and discussions with trusted colleagues about the best means of helping couples struggling to recover from an affair. Since its first edition, published in 2007, the book has guided this recovery process for tens of thousands of couples and received the Self-Help Seal of Merit from the Association for Behavioral and Cognitive Therapies. We also published a companion book for mental health professionals and other counselors helping couples recover from an affair in 2009, and since then we've trained thousands of professionals in promoting affair recovery using these resources.

In the 16 years since the first edition, the path toward recovery has remained largely unchanged, although the nature of couple relationships and affairs has evolved. Relationships that don't fit the pattern of different-sex married couples have become more public and more common. Emerging technologies enable secret involvement with someone outside the relationship easier to pursue. Use of social media increases the likelihood that the trauma of an affair will become public knowledge in ways that can make recovery more difficult. This second edition reflects these developments in direct and intentional ways.

The case vignettes interwoven throughout this edition reflect a much broader diversity of couples in relationship patterns, ethnicity, and culture. They're drawn from our research and clinical practice. In all instances, names and identifying information have been changed. Consistent with our wish to represent as many readers as possible, we typically use "they" or "them" to refer to a person whose gender is unspecified or not relevant to the issue being addressed.

Along the way, several people provided special encouragement and assistance facilitating completion of this work. We thank our editors at The Guilford Press—especially Kitty Moore, whose steadfast encouragement and patience never wavered despite the passing of numerous deadlines. Kitty and her colleague, Chris Benton, provided keen insights that helped to guide revisions to the first edition. The support and encouragement of our colleagues, students, and clients have been vital. Our thinking was frequently sharpened by lively discussions about relationship injuries, forgiveness, and strategies for promoting recovery.

We're particularly indebted to Emily Carrino, an aspiring and gifted clinical psychologist from the University of North Carolina, whose unique perspectives and thoughtful comments are reflected in important ways in this revised edition. Emily brought a fresh viewpoint and considerable wisdom about the changing nature of relationships, emerging technologies, and special considerations of nontraditional couples that significantly enhanced this second edition of the book.

Above all, we are profoundly grateful for the faithful encouragement of our own partners, without whom we could not have completed this book. Your understanding and loving support throughout both the first and second editions sustained and strengthened us during times we needed it most. Thank you for sharing with us the best of what an intimate relationship can offer.

Introduction

Erin sat motionless in front of the laptop. She didn't know how long she'd been there and just stared at the screen in disbelief. "I can't wait to be with you again. You've changed my life—I've finally found my soulmate." Someone named Amber had written those words to her husband. Erin could hardly absorb what she'd read. Her brain had turned off, and she felt numb. In one brief moment, her life had changed forever. She felt utterly destroyed and betrayed.

If you've discovered that your partner has had an affair, you probably know how Erin feels. Waves of painful emotion can make it hard to put one foot in front of the other and just go about your daily business. The barrage of conflicting thoughts about how this could have happened—and the haunting flashbacks and questions about what actually did happen—may be so distracting that you can't get anything done. And when you even think about how you're *supposed* to react as a betrayed partner, the only solutions that come to mind are the types of soap opera clichés you've always laughed at. So what *are* you supposed to do? How do you make sense of this and put your life back together?

We wrote this book to walk you through an agonizing time in your life and lead you to the answers that are best for you. The best answers for you may not prove to be the best answers for your partner—and certainly not for the couple down the street. But each of you has a chance to move on in a healthy way if you put in the hard work.

Moving on in a healthy way means recovering *personally* from the affair so that you can pursue the future you want. It means knowing enough about what happened and *why* it happened to make a wise decision about whether to stay together or part. It means protecting yourself from being hurt again without carrying the backbreaking—and heartbreaking—burden of anger and suspicion or guilt and shame for the rest of your life.

In this book you'll read about a process that has helped many couples move on from an affair in a healthy way. We'll provide you with a clear but flexible set of steps, based on our treatment for infidelity, which has been studied scientifically, a treatment that grew out of many decades of our collective clinical experience and that we've taught to other therapists for many years. All three of us are clinical psychologists and therapists who specialize in working with couples having relationship difficulties, infidelity being one of our major areas of work. We're also university professors and researchers who conduct systematic research on these issues. We've written numerous articles and conducted frequent workshops for therapists in the United States and abroad on helping couples who are struggling to recover from an affair. All of this experience across these various areas has gone into the recovery process you'll read about here.

Why should you undertake this work, especially when you're feeling so beaten down or feel so helpless from the trauma of the affair? ***Because the issues you're wrestling with right now won't just go away with time.*** The intensity of your pain might decrease somewhat with time, but that won't address important issues that are essential for moving forward. If you simply try to wait out the pain, or tackle problems and issues in the wrong order, you can easily make decisions you'll later regret. You can also end up with unresolved hurt and anger. Right after an affair is revealed, the most important tasks are to find a way to cope with the emotional turmoil and to know how to get through the day with your partner without making things worse or letting the rest of your life fall apart. After taking care of the immediate aspects of your life, you can then benefit from taking a close look at your partner, yourself, and your history together so that you can figure out what made your relationship vulnerable to an affair and how you could change things in the future so that this relationship or a future one is on more solid ground.

This *is* important work you should do, and the best way to emerge whole after an affair. Following the process described in this book can help you develop a new understanding of yourself and your partner. You may emerge with a new view of what it means to be in a committed relationship and what a healthy partner and partnership look like. And, though you may not believe it right now, if this turns out to be what you want, you could end up with a relationship that's potentially even stronger and better than it was before the affair.

Who Can Use This Book?

■ This book is for anyone who has experienced an affair. Currently about 25% of men and 15% of women engage in sexual infidelity at some point in their lives—and nearly 45% of men and 35% of women when emotional (nonsexual) affairs are included. Moreover, there are many ways that partners can be unfaithful or cross the line that don't fit neatly into categories and can leave you confused and asking, "Was that an affair? I know it feels terrible; I feel betrayed—but I don't even know exactly why or what to call it."

■ An affair involves becoming romantically, emotionally, or sexually involved with someone else in a way that violates important expectations or standards of your relationship. That is, another person or other people are being brought into your relationship in ways that should have been reserved for just your own intimate relationship—boundaries have been crossed. For many couples, those boundaries might be defined as **not** being sexually involved with another person or **not** becoming too emotionally intimate with someone else. But what if your partner is just fantasizing about someone and doesn't even tell the other person—is that a violation? What if your partner is interacting online in a chat room with someone they don't ever meet in person? Or visiting pornographic websites secretly? Depending on the couple and what they expect of each other as partners, all of these circumstances might involve crossing important boundaries and feel like a betrayal. To some couples, however, some of these actions (watching pornography, for example) might be considered acceptable and are within the bounds of what is okay to do in your relationship. Either way, your relationship boundaries are *your* relationship boundaries—regardless of what other couples are doing (or *not* doing).

So, as technology expands and as individuals explore a wide range of relationships, the ways that partners might cross important boundaries expand as well, no matter what words you use to define them—an affair, infidelity, betrayal, outside involvement, one-night stand, or something else, depending on its duration or intensity. Or, none of these words might seem to quite fit, but you recognize that your partner has "crossed the line" in some important way that feels terrible and has you confused or doubting your partner and your relationship. Often this happens when some kind of deceit is involved.

■ This book is for you if you're in a committed relationship, whether you're married or not. Your legal status doesn't define your commitment to each other, the expectations you have of each other, or the boundaries you expect between you as a couple and other people. Likewise, the principles underlying the importance of boundaries play out regardless of your gender or sexual orientation, although every couple has its own definition of those boundaries. Some couples agree to boundaries that extend beyond just the two of them; that is, they might agree to a nonmonogamous relationship that involves other people in a romantic or sexual way. Even so, there are typically expectations about what these various relationships should look like, and those boundaries can be violated.

■ You stand to gain from this book whether the affair was just revealed or you've been struggling with it for some time. Even if you just found out about the affair, it might have ended long ago or only recently, or it might be ongoing. In many instances, the pain and confusion are just as intense, and the process you need to follow is fundamentally the same in these various situations.

■ The book will help you recover whether you're the injured partner (the one who did *not* have the affair) or the involved partner (the one who did). When we say "you" here and in the rest of this book, most of the time we mean the injured partner. Our work has shown that injured partners are *generally* more traumatized by an affair than involved partners, and therefore they're more likely to seek help. But at times we'll also address the person who had the affair (and we'll make clear when we're doing so), as well as the two of you as a couple. You stand the best chance of emerging whole and healthy when you both gain a full understanding of what happened.

■ You can benefit from doing the work in this book whether you do it alone or with your partner. If your partner reads it too, even if the two of you work through it separately, *you* will be the beneficiary. Participants in affairs need to be honest with themselves about whether they're ready to end all involvement with the outside person. They need to figure out how to express care for their partners once the affair is over, as well as remorse. It's important that they understand why they ended up getting involved in an affair. If your partner explores these issues, trust and intimacy might grow between you again.

How Should You Use This Book?

Ideally, both you and your partner will read each chapter and work through the recovery process we describe. You can do much of the suggested work separately, but some of it involves having conversations or engaging in activities together that will help you move forward. Still, we know that reality is rarely ideal, and you may end up working through this book alone for different reasons. Maybe your partner is one of those people who really don't like "self-help" books. Or perhaps your partner refuses to discuss what's happened. Or possibly you've already ended your relationship with your partner because of an affair, but you want to explore the experience on your own. That's a wise move, because there's plenty of research (including our own) that suggests that if traumatic relationship events such as an affair aren't addressed adequately, their negative impact could affect future relationships. If you have children with your partner, reading this book may help you resolve lingering resentments that might otherwise spill over into your co-parenting relationship and negatively affect your children.

Whether for these reasons or any others you plan to use this book on your own, your personal insights and increased understanding can put you in a better position to decide what to do about the future of your relationship if you're still with your partner. Moreover, once you learn to think about the affair and approach your life differently, you can change your relationship to an extent even if your partner isn't involved in making the same efforts. Although two people working together to make changes are often more effective than one, even one is better than none. And, even if your relationship ends, you might still learn something helpful for your own growth. So read this book for yourself and for your relationship— current or future. If you're involved in individual counseling while reading this book, share what you're reading with your counselor and together explore how this material applies to you.

We've presented the chapters in the order that has been most helpful to the couples we've counseled, and the chapters generally build on each other, but if certain questions seem particularly important to you, go ahead and read in whatever order you wish.

What Will You Gain?

Based on the couples we've ushered through this recovery process, we know that your first likely challenge is to deal with the initial devastation by avoiding further damage to your relationship and managing essential tasks in the home.

Part I is about coping with the immediate trauma after finding out about the affair. It can help you:

- Deal with intense feelings—your own and your partner's.
- Communicate about extremely difficult topics.
- Decide how to go on with your daily routine, from managing chores and finances to parenting.
- Figure out how to keep living together while you regroup (should you sleep in the same bed? Have sex?)—and under what circumstances an immediate separation makes sense.
- Establish boundaries and limits with the outside affair person (the one with whom the involved partner had the affair)—who may not want to end the affair.
- Determine how much, if anything, to share with others about the affair—including your children, family members, or close friends.
- Take care of yourself even if it seems like a low priority, including getting help from friends and seeing your doctor when you need to.

Once you and your partner have restored some equilibrium to your relationship, Part II will help you examine the various factors that might have made your relationship vulnerable to an affair. It can help you:

- Look clearly at your relationship over time—whether it's fulfilled your dreams, how it's changed, whether its foundations were shaken, and by what.

- Understand the characteristics and events that led one of you to have an affair.

- Understand what "infidelity" really means—and how boundaries can get crossed, even without any intention of hurting anyone.

- Recognize how your environment, events, and other people helped set the stage for the affair or made it more likely.

- Understand how the injured partner can unintentionally contribute to a relationship's vulnerability—without being responsible for the involved partner's decision to have an affair.

- Avoid the temptation to be content with incomplete or partly accurate explanations just to avoid delving deeply into difficult topics.

- Arrive at a coherent picture or "narrative" of the affair that makes sense.

Part III guides you in making good decisions about moving forward—either separately or together. It can help you:

- Consider what it means to "move on" and how to get past disabling hurt feelings.

- Anticipate and deal with setbacks, whether together or apart.

- Continue strengthening your relationship and minimizing future risks if you've decided to stay together.

Although we don't presume to know what decisions you'll make down the road, we're confident that working through this book can help to lead you through a healthy process as you make the journey. We hope it will help ease the pain and uncertainty along the way. Right now, just understanding what's happened, figuring out how to get through the day, and hurting less are important goals. So, let's get started.

PART I

How Do We Stop Hurting?

1

What's Happening to Us?

"It's been three weeks since I found out. In some ways, it feels like it just happened, and at the same time it feels like this is going on forever. Just when I start to feel like I'm holding it together, I fall apart again. I know I'm jumpy and irritable. I can't concentrate, I can't sleep, and I'm forgetting things at home and at work. We talk, we avoid each other—it doesn't matter. Nothing's working. This isn't the person I married. I don't trust what I thought we had, and I can't imagine trusting again in the future. Nothing makes sense anymore."

What's Going On with Me?

If you've just learned that your partner has had an affair, you're struggling with one of the most traumatic experiences a person can face. (If you're the person who had the affair, you're likely also struggling, and we'll talk about that later in the chapter.) There are all kinds of traumatic events—from floods or plane crashes to infidelity. Any of these can be overwhelming. But natural disasters and mechanical failure are unintentional and typically unavoidable. A partner's affair results from deliberate decisions by your *partner*—the one person who's supposed to love and care for you, protect you from the rest of the world, and treat you with respect, dignity, and honesty. For many people, few betrayals can be more hurtful and disruptive.

Understanding the impact of traumatic events and how most people recover from them can help you develop a larger picture of what's happening to you and your partner and what's likely to happen to you both in the future. So, first, what *is* a traumatic event?

> 🖋 A trauma is a major negative event or set of events that destroys important assumptions or fundamental beliefs about the world or specific people—in this case, your partner and your relationship.
>
> Traumatic events disrupt all parts of your life—your thoughts, feelings, and behaviors.

You assumed that your relationship would be safe and that your well-being would be uppermost in your partner's mind, both when you were together and when you were apart. You trusted that your partner valued you and your relationship. You expected honesty—that no large parts of your partner's life would be hidden from you. Finally, you expected your partner to honor commitments you made to each other—whether stated out loud or just understood.

So what is it about an affair that makes it so painful? If you're like most people, it's particularly upsetting if your partner violates important boundaries in your relationship that you agreed or assumed would be respected. You might have talked about these boundaries (for example, "I don't feel comfortable with you talking to your ex-girlfriend"), or they seemed so obvious to you that you assumed you and partner would honor them (such as "You can't have sex with anyone except your partner; that's a given and no discussion is needed"). Whether you ever stated them explicitly or not, you (and all couples) create boundaries around your relationship that determine how you interact with others—for example, "*This* part of our life is just for the two of us; no one crosses *this* boundary into our relationship. We don't do *this* with other people." Where you and your partner set the boundaries might be different from where other couples set theirs. In affairs, boundaries that are crossed typically involve a couple's sex life (for example, kissing and intimately touching someone else) or romantic connections with others (for example, going on dates with other people when you're in an exclusive relationship or treating a work friend in an overly special way). So, if one of these boundaries has been crossed, of course you're likely to feel betrayed and upset.

For some couples and perhaps for you, it's also a violation if your partner *feels* particularly intimate with another person, even if it's just "inside their head" and not acted upon (for example, fantasizing and having strong feelings about another person). The main point is: *If you're experiencing that your partner has had an affair or has been unfaithful, in most instances this means that your partner has disrespected important boundaries around your relationship in one way or another.* Boundaries protect us and give us safety. And crossing the boundary is made worse if your partner tries to hide, minimize, or even lie about what has happened because it makes restoring trust even more difficult.

It's important that both of you be clear on what boundary violations have occurred. Throughout the book, we'll discuss different types of boundaries that partners sometimes cross that can throw their relationships into chaos; most likely, some of those will ring true for you. It's also important for both of you to understand how the violation came about; an explanation of "it just happened" won't protect you and your relationship from similar betrayals in the future.

Whereas understanding the betrayal of infidelity and how it happened is crucial, often this isn't enough because the impact goes far beyond those specific betrayals. Becoming aware that your partner has betrayed you might call into question other important assumptions you have about your partner and your relationship. How many of the following thoughts have you had since learning of your partner's affair?

- You question previous beliefs about your partner—for example, no longer viewing your partner as caring or trustworthy.

- Your beliefs about the relationship are shattered—for example, you no longer view your relationship as a source of support or fulfillment.

- You adopt extreme, negative explanations for your partner's behavior—for example, thinking your partner *wanted* to hurt you deeply.

- You fear that other betrayals may remain hidden or lie ahead.

- You have the sense that your relationship is beyond your control—that you have little influence over what happens between you and your partner.

Learning about your partner's affair may even lead you to question beliefs or feelings about yourself—for example:

- You feel foolish or ashamed for not having recognized warning signs earlier.

- You don't trust your own judgment, or you blame yourself for not listening to concerns about your partner expressed by family or friends.

- You wonder about your own attractiveness or whether you fell short as a partner in important ways.

Not surprisingly, people are at high risk for developing significant depression and anxiety after experiencing a betrayal such as an affair, just as they would after any significant loss. Affairs bring about many losses— loss of safety and predictability, loss of dreams for your relationship and perhaps for your future, loss of innocence, loss of trust. These are on top of the loss of something special and unique that you two shared exclusively: sex, romance, and your innermost thoughts and feelings.

You might experience a wide range of other negative feelings as well, from anger to anxiety and fear or even guilt and shame. Anger is a common reaction to believing you've been treated unfairly, and affairs feel extremely unfair. Does your anger make sense? Absolutely. Fear and anxiety arise when your world feels unsafe and unpredictable. A partner's affair breaks down all the protective walls, and suddenly nothing feels safe or predictable anymore.

Guilt usually results when you think you're to blame or have done something wrong. In trying to make sense of a partner's affair, some people conclude, "At some level, it must be my fault. I must have done something to cause it to happen." Those feelings, too, are understandable, but make no mistake about it: *Your partner's affair isn't your fault*. In Part II of this book, we'll help you explore your own role in creating your relationship with your partner. But your partner has to take responsibility for their own individual behavior—and that includes the decision to have an affair.

Which of these feelings have you already experienced? You may experience some of the following later on, if you haven't already.

- You feel strong, overwhelming emotions such as anger, depression, or anxiety.
- On the other hand, at times you feel nothing at all, just numb or flat.
- You feel profoundly vulnerable and unsafe.
- Your feelings are unpredictable, possibly changing daily or hourly.
- You're confused about what you feel and about what you want either now or in the future.

On a fundamental level, an affair throws your normal emotional state into total disarray. Your feelings might change from one minute to the next. Or they might be so jumbled together that you don't know what you feel. Maybe you're not really feeling much of anything—and think there must be something wrong with you because you're not. Research suggests that a trauma is often followed by an initial sense of numbness, possibly as a way of protecting ourselves from being overwhelmed by intense feelings. In most cases, those feelings surface at some later point. How many of the following descriptions fit with your own experience?

- You have flashbacks in which you reexperience painful feelings, memories, or images from the affair. (We'll discuss these further in Chapter 2.)
- You feel as though your emotions can overwhelm you or are out of your control.
- You have periods of numbness when you don't feel much of anything at all.

If you're one of those people who *is* experiencing a lot of strong emotion, your behavior is also likely to be out of character or at times even chaotic. When you can no longer trust or believe what you've always taken as a given, you're not likely to act the way you used to either. You might find yourself shouting at a grocery store clerk for no good reason or showing up unannounced at your partner's office to talk—only to change your mind and leave abruptly. Or you may find yourself driving toward the outside affair person's home or place of business, not entirely clear about what you would do or say if you were to confront that person. You might even find that, at times, you act outside of your own value system, which can be confusing to you and make matters worse; for example, research suggests that some people become physically aggressive toward their partner or the outside person after they find out about an affair. While anger is common, such aggression is obviously problematic and potentially dangerous. If you're struggling with managing your anger, you may want to jump ahead to the guidelines for handling strong emotions in Chapter 3.

Which of the following describe some of your own experiences?

- You act disoriented—for example, staring off into space or wandering about with no apparent purpose or direction.

- You retreat emotionally or physically—for example, withdrawing into long silences or avoiding interaction and finding places to be alone.

- You repeatedly ask for an explanation of your partner's behavior—for example, "How could you do this?"

- You seek revenge—for example, attacking your partner verbally or physically, destroying your partner's property, or harming their relationships with others.

- You try to reassure yourself—for example, initiating frequent and intense sexual encounters with your partner in an attempt to make up for your partner's previous complaints about your sexual relationship.

Your usual daily routines with your partner may also be called into question. Are you really going to get up and make coffee for someone who betrayed you? You used to give each other a quick kiss when one of you left in the morning—but now that feels awkward. Or perhaps now when your partner touches you, you cringe as it brings back painful memories, or instead maybe you want to sink into an embrace, trying to feel connected again. Should you still go out to dinner together with friends? If so, are you cold and distant, or do you pretend to be the happy couple while inside you just want to scream? Behaviors you took for granted, which had become routine and almost automatic, now seem awkward, disgusting, or unsafe.

The bottom line is that a partner's affair is a big deal. *It's traumatic.* It involves violations of boundaries and core assumptions about your partner, your relationship, and perhaps even yourself. You can anticipate a wide variety of feelings, most of them negative. And at times you're going to say and do things that just aren't like you. It's miserable. It feels awful. But it's also a normal reaction to what's happened. And our research and clinical work with couples strongly suggest that if you go through the recovery process in a healthy manner, these feelings won't remain as strong as they are right now, and they won't be there all the time. Things can get better.

What's Happening to Our Relationship?

Part of what's happening to you as a couple right now is a direct result of the turmoil that's going on with each of you individually. Let's face it: No matter how well your partner might be managing their own feelings, your relationship isn't likely to go well when you're still struggling with the initial trauma of finding out about the affair. You're not likely to express yourself effectively. You're probably not able to listen in a caring way to your partner's views. You may find it difficult to work together on even routine tasks such as paying bills together, making decisions about the children, dealing with a car that needs repair, or the hundreds of other mundane chores involved in having a committed partnership. And when these tasks don't get done, the negative consequences of neglecting them can bring additional stress. The phone company threatens to disconnect your phone; one of the kids gets into trouble at school; the rattle under the hood turns into a major engine overhaul with no money to pay for it.

All that can happen even when your partner is handling their own feelings reasonably well. Chances are they aren't. Independent of what you're feeling, your partner is probably struggling with their own turmoil. Right now, you may have too much of your own hurt or anger to be very sympathetic. That's understandable. But at some point, if you want to be able to interact more effectively, you're going to need a better understanding of what your partner is experiencing. Reading the material on pages 23–27, where we speak to your partner, might be helpful when you decide you want to gain more of this understanding. But for now, just consider that your partner is probably wrestling with difficult feelings too—possibly including confusion and uncertainty about the future, anxiety about your relationship, aloneness, hurt, anger, guilt, or shame. In fact, even if *you* are managing your own feelings well, there's a good chance your relationship would still be feeling crazy because of what's going on with your partner right now.

Mix together these two factors—your own turmoil and your partner's—and you have the perfect formula for chaos. Just when you feel able to talk constructively, your partner won't. And just when your partner feels able to approach you or respond constructively, you can't. Moreover, whatever feelings either one of you is struggling with at any given moment can trigger equally intense and difficult feelings in the other.

To understand why this happens, it's helpful to think of your interactions as serving three functions—communication, protection, and restoration—each of which is made more difficult by the trauma of the affair:

1. It's too hard for your partner to hear what you feel has to be said. You want your partner to understand the awful feelings and confusion caused by the affair. Those feelings are intense, sometimes exceeding your ability to express them well. And if your partner cares for you at all, hearing you express these feelings will be uncomfortable or even painful—especially if they're struggling with their own guilt or shame. After all, your partner was the source of your trauma, so hearing you talk about it may increase their own distress or impulse to pull back or stop listening when you continue to express your feelings. At that point you're likely to feel unheard, and you're going to crank up the volume. But then a person who already feels on the defensive or overwhelmed by the intensity of your feelings is going to pull back even further or possibly lash out in response, and you're going to feel even less heard and less understood. It's a vicious cycle of wanting to be understood and instead feeling less and less heard by your partner.

2. The need to feel safe often means trying to protect yourselves from each other. In addition to wanting to be understood, both you and your partner want to feel safe. But you can't feel emotionally safe when you're afraid you might be hurt again. You've probably heard of the "fight-or-flight" response to feeling threatened. When you choose to "fight" in response to danger, you go on the offensive and keep others away by threatening to do them harm. So, in an effort to protect yourself, you may sometimes punish your partner verbally: "How could you be so cruel? I hate you." "Where was your integrity? Just wait until I tell the children."

Forcefully pursuing control can be another way to "fight" your way to safety: "You're never going anywhere again without my knowing where and without checking in." "You can't be trusted; I want our bank accounts signed over to me." Physical aggression can be still another way of seeking safety, even when initiated by someone who's physically smaller and less powerful. It's a way of saying "Stay away from me unless you want to get hurt." However, fighting in a relationship is rarely an effective way to ensure safety and can lead to counterattacks from your partner.

Some partners who need safety choose "flight" instead of "fight," retreating physically by demanding separate bedrooms or separate living quarters or retreating verbally—withdrawing into silence and refusing to interact. Other kinds of retreat can be more subtle. For example, some couples end up leading a civil life together but really talk only about superficial things, ignoring more difficult issues and never restoring an intimate relationship.

What can make this all very complicated and confusing is that your efforts to create safety can backfire. For example, when your questioning triggers an angry defense from your partner, each of you may be trying to feel safer but instead end up feeling more threatened. Or there may be times when you've pulled back into silence and your partner tries to reassure you, but your partner's caring behaviors feel too scary for you, and you use anger to push your partner away.

3. **It's not just the thought that counts in efforts to restore the relationship—it's applying the right strategies at the right time.** Each of you may be trying in your own way to restore your relationship, but these efforts just aren't working. Those who have been involved in an affair often try to repair their relationship by convincing the injured partner that the affair didn't really mean anything or that they're totally committed to the relationship but just didn't realize it before. Injured partners sometimes try to restore their relationship by trying to push thoughts of the affair completely out of their minds or by finding out "why" the partner had the affair. Such attempts may ultimately reflect the right goal, but they can fall short unless they are well thought through:

■ **Is this the right move?** Sometimes efforts backfire, doing more damage instead of restoring the relationship. For example, trying to promote closeness by insisting that you and your partner do everything together may instead make your partner feel suffocated and desperate to escape.

■ **Is it the right time?** Even fundamentally good strategies have to be implemented in the right order. Insistence on having long discussions about what led to the affair, while ultimately a crucial part of restoring long-term security to your relationship, won't be constructive if one of you still feels deeply misunderstood or too emotionally vulnerable to the other. Deciding when to have difficult discussions can be critical to listening well and hearing what your partner has to say.

Fortunately, both ineffective strategies and poor timing often can be avoided. In fact, the whole purpose of this book is to provide you with effective ways of communicating, reestablishing safety, and restoring individual and relationship security—and implementing these strategies in a sequence and time frame that are more likely to be successful.

Do We Have a Future Together?

This question may be the most important issue you're facing right now. Can you and your partner truly recover? Can you restore a trusting, loving relationship and move on together to bring each other joy and enrich one another's life?

Our answer to this is "Maybe." We can tell you that among legally married couples in which one member has recently learned of the partner's affair, only a minority go on to divorce. Most, approximately 60–75%, remain married. Among those couples who stay together, many go on to restore a loving and secure relationship. But some couples struggling to recover from an affair remain married yet continue feeling hurt, distrustful, and very unhappy. It's also not clear to what extent affairs lead to breakups for couples who aren't legally married; there's little research on these couples, and moreover, they don't have to deal with the legal complications of ending a marriage. So it might be easier to end these relationships from a practical and legal standpoint, although not necessarily easier emotionally. For couples who have relationship agreements that may allow for romantic and sexual involvement with others (for example, some people in polyamorous or "open" relationships), boundaries still exist ("You can sleep with other people, but don't fall in love with them") and can be crossed (secretively or not), although there are no data on whether those relationships are more likely to end after an affair. The important message is that what will happen with your relationship as you move forward isn't predetermined; this is up to the two of you, and there are lots of factors to consider in making those decisions.

At this point you're undoubtedly struggling with so many confusing emotions that you don't even know whether you both *want* to stay together. That's fine. Just keep in mind that eventually you'll have to figure out what you both want in addition to what's possible. As to whether you can restore a secure relationship, we emphasized in the Introduction that **couples need to accomplish three critical tasks:**

1. Find ways to manage and minimize the painful emotions
2. Come to understand how the affair came about
3. Reach an explicit, informed decision about how to move forward

If you've just recently found out about the affair, you and your partner need to concentrate on task number one, finding ways of surviving the immediate crisis, because it's difficult to start exploring what happened when you're preoccupied by confusing and troubling emotions and don't know how to interact with your partner anymore. This requires managing strong feelings to address a lot of practical decisions in addition to simply taking better care of yourself: Should you touch each other, sleep together, make love? How do you handle anger? How do you start talking about the affair without making things worse? What do you do when your daily routine is disrupted by repeated memories or "flashbacks" of the affair? How do you deal with the outside affair person, and what will you tell your children and others, if anything?

Once you've addressed these issues, you've cleared a path for determining what happened that led you to this situation. What placed your relationship at risk for an affair? What has to happen so you can eliminate or reduce those risks in the future? How can you assure yourselves and each other of your commitment to pursuing these changes? *Answering these questions is difficult, without a doubt, but lies at the very heart of recovery.* You'll have to be willing to look closely at your relationship, at things that were happening outside your relationship, at your partner and even yourself if you want to get more complete answers. As we said earlier, no one is responsible for their partner's infidelity, but it's important to find out whether you contributed to an environment that makes either partner susceptible to an affair.

> Difficult conversations with Damien led Liz to conclude that there were some early warning signs of Damien's emotional withdrawal before he had his affair, but at the time these felt too threatening to Liz to confront directly. To eliminate the danger of the same pattern happening again, Liz ultimately agreed that she would ask Damien what was going on with him if she thought he was withdrawing again, and Damien agreed that he would address her concerns directly and honestly. Both agreed to work at expressing and responding to such concerns without anger. Each pledged to protect their relationship from situations that had placed them at risk for an affair in the past, and they committed to making their marriage their top priority. But it took time and effort to get to this point. The reward, both felt, was worth it all: they reestablished the emotional security that's critical to an intimate relationship.

With that emotional security in place, Liz and Damien were able to reconcile, as many other couples are too. But the goal of doing this work is to reach a healthy, informed decision about how to move on, and that doesn't necessarily mean reconciling or staying together. People can work through this recovery process by restoring their relationship to its previous form, by changing and strengthening it, or by ending it. By "moving on" we mean that each of you will be able to move beyond focusing almost exclusively on the affair, and you'll voluntarily stop punishing each other. Instead, you'll each be able to redirect your efforts toward an emotionally satisfying and productive life, either together or apart. This affair will never be forgotten. But it will no longer dominate your lives.

The step-by-step process for recovering from an affair that we outline in this book has helped many couples move forward in a healthier way. Most—about 70%—choose to rebuild their relationship. Many of these—nearly half—restore an intimate relationship that's stronger than it was before the affair. Other couples find this process helpful but may continue to struggle with individual or relationship problems that were present long before the affair—such as sexual difficulties, substance use, depression, or other emotional or behavioral difficulties. Some individuals work through the process outlined here and decide to end their relationship and move on separately. Among these, many discover that their improved understanding of themselves and others allows them to develop stronger, deeper relationships in the future, perhaps including a new partner.

Whether you move on together or separately is something we encourage you to decide later, after you've finished obtaining a more complete understanding of what's happened. If you and your partner have already reached a long-term decision about your relationship, that's okay. But we'd still suggest that you hold the decision open and revisit it from time to time as you gain new information and understanding.

In reaching any decision, it's important to understand what was happening with both of you that set the stage for an affair. If you feel ready to consider some of what your partner might be experiencing in all of this at present, read on. If you don't feel receptive to that right now, put the book away for a while and come back to it when you're ready. Ultimately, to move on with your own recovery process, you'll want to continue from here and understand your partner better. It's not uncommon that our most intimate and rewarding relationships are also the source of our deepest hurt and disappointment. However, recovery from even the most profound relationship heartaches *can* occur. The process we've outlined in this book can help.

For the Involved Partner

"I know I've screwed up; that's not the problem. The problem is, I don't know how to make it better again. I'm doing everything I know how to get us back on track. But nothing seems to work. She wants to talk about the affair, and I don't. Talking about it just seems to get her more upset. But if I don't talk about it, she thinks I'm trying to hide something, or that I don't understand how hurt she is, or I just *don't care enough to work on it. Sure I care. That's why I'm trying to avoid these awful arguments we get into every time she asks questions about how I cheated on her. We go over and over the same old stuff. I don't know if there's anything I can do at this point to make things better."*

How Can I Be Helpful?

If your partner has recently learned about your affair, and you're reading this book, you've already taken a critical step toward being helpful.

🖋 The most important things you can communicate to your partner right now are that:

—You want to understand what's happening to each of you.

—You're willing to take a hard look at how this affair came about.

—You want to figure out the best way to move on.

That's what this book is all about. It's going to take patience, commitment to the entire process, and lots of hard work. But continuing to read through the next few pages is an important first step.

You may not be willing to do this. Some people who've had an affair already have their bags packed and have one foot out the door. Others apologize and take their punishment but don't really want to do any additional work to make the relationship right again: "I've ended it; what more do you want?" And even if you *are* willing, you and your partner might not be able to make your relationship survive despite patience, commitment, and hard work. Affairs happen for all kinds of reasons, to all kinds of people in all kinds of circumstances. So we couldn't begin to tell you at this point whether your relationship can—or should—be saved.

As mentioned above, some couples stay together; some don't. Of the couples that stay together, some go on to build a better and stronger relationship; others stay together but remain hurt, angry, distrustful, and generally miserable. The same is true for couples who break up or divorce following an affair. For partners who've done the work to know themselves better, understand their own needs and vulnerabilities, and find a way of placing their own or their partner's affair into a bigger life picture, moving on separately can sometimes permit new, healthier relationships to develop. But for partners who divorce out of anger, confusion, or just not knowing a process for making good decisions, life after a divorce can continue to feel as hurtful or as empty as the relationship did following the affair.

How can you help the recovery process? For now, we invite you to take three very important steps. None may be easy. Each might be more difficult than the one listed just before it.

1. **Work at understanding your partner's experience.** If you haven't done so already, go back and read this chapter from the beginning. You're going to read about how your affair has impacted your partner. Reading this might be uncomfortable or even painful. But an important message you'll be communicating to your partner is this: "I want to understand how you're feeling right now. Sometimes it's hard for me to listen to you when you're so angry, or to ask about your feelings when you've pulled back into silence. But I do want to understand so I'll know better how to respond."

2. **Commit to a recovery *process*.** You and your partner don't need to decide right now whether to stay in this relationship for the long term. Instead, we encourage you to commit the necessary time and effort to understand the impact of your affair, explore the various reasons for it, and then decide with your partner how you can each move on to a full and enriching life—together or separately.

3. **Avoid doing more damage.** As obvious as this step sounds, it can be the most difficult of all. Right now, both you and your partner might have some very strong feelings. It's easy to escalate into heated arguments. It's easy to be misunderstood. It's hard to avoid falling into the trap of attacks and counterattacks. In the next three chapters, we're going to give you some concrete steps for avoiding doing more damage. But for now, specific things to do are:

- *Be patient.* If you expect recovery to be quick, you're going to be frustrated. If you expect your partner to get over it, you're going to be disappointed. And if you require yourself to be perfect in your own responses, you're going to feel disillusioned.

- *Be truthful.* Continued dishonesty, deception, and half-truths ultimately will be more destructive than your affair itself. This doesn't mean that you have to disclose every detail of your affair; that can also be destructive. But if you say something, be sure it's the truth. If your partner asks you a question and you're not yet willing to answer, just say so: "I know this is important to you. And I don't want any more secrets or dishonesty. But I'm not able to talk about this with you yet."

■ *Be trusting.* Specifically, trust the process. We're confident that if each of you commits to the process we're going to take you through in this book, you're each going to end up in a better place—less hurt, less angry, and better equipped to move on and lead a happier life again.

What about Me?

Marcus had been feeling hurt and neglected by Lucia, who seemed to be completely wrapped up in their new baby and too tired to even think about sex. He thought visiting a sexually explicit chat room on the internet would be a safe outlet and never expected to arrange to meet someone in person. It just felt so good to be wanted, and a small part of him felt angry and justified in his behavior. Later, when he looked back on the experience, he felt dirty and ashamed. How could he do that to his new family? What had come over him?

Your partner's probably not the only one who feels misunderstood. There's a good chance you do too. You might be feeling one or more of the following:

Confused. "How did I get into this mess? How do I get out of it? How do I make things right again?"

Hurt. "Can't she see that I didn't intend to hurt her? What more can I say? Why can't she accept my apology?"

Angry. "It's not all me. Yes, I'm the one who had the affair. But this relationship was far from perfect, and he had a lot to do with that. I'm tired of taking all the blame and punishment for this mess. Enough is enough."

Guilty or ashamed. "I deserve whatever I get. I want her to forgive me and move on, but that's probably too much to hope for and certainly too much to ask. I can't stand to hear her talk about her feelings about the affair; it makes me feel terrible, like I'm a heartless jerk or something. I wish she'd just let it be."

Alone. "If I thought I was alone before, that was nothing compared to how I feel now. Right now I have no one. I don't know how much longer I can go on this way."

Uncertain. "I just don't know for sure what I want. I know having an affair wasn't the right answer to whatever problems or feelings I was having before. But I'm not sure what the right answer is or how to find it."

During the process you're about to undertake, you'll be addressing difficult feelings and questions that you and your partner both have—whether you're working together as a couple or separately by yourself. Early in this process, your partner might have difficulty listening to what you need or how you feel. Your partner might feel that your relationship is already unbalanced and you've been focusing mostly on what *you* want. As you move through this process and are able to listen to your partner's hurt and pain, often your partner can start to do the same in hearing from you.

We encourage you to be patient and truthful and to trust in the process. We're not going to ask you and your partner to do this all at once. We're going to take you through the process step by step. However, as therapists we've experienced the remarkable strengths that both partners can bring to a damaged relationship when they're given a process for doing so. **We've worked with many couples whose relationships actually ended up stronger, more faithful, and more personally fulfilling for both partners after the affair.** We hope this may be possible for you; but if you need to end the relationship, we'll try to help you do this constructively.

So what's next? Whether you're the injured or the involved partner, do the exercises on the following pages. If you're reading this book alone and want your partner's involvement, we encourage you to approach your partner and say something like the following: "I know this is really difficult, but I want us to find a way of working through this situation. I found a book that I think could help us. I've read the first chapter, and much of it makes sense to me. Please read through the first chapter and let me know when you're finished. I need to know whether we can commit to a process that can help us work together to move forward." Find a way to express your wish as an invitation or request, not as a threat or demand. What's important is that the message comes out of your sincere concern for your relationship. Neither of you needs to commit to anything other than the wish that you'll each be able to recover and move on toward a fruitful and happy life.

If your partner still won't join you in working through the recovery process outlined in this book, there are three important things you can still do:

1. **Work through this book on your own.** Begin by working through this first set of exercises to reach for your own personal recovery. You could end up restoring this relationship through your own understanding of what's happened and how to prevent it from happening again. Or, if you end this relationship, your own recovery will leave you better able to pursue a satisfying life single or as part of a new couple.

2. **Don't give up hope.** Your own personal recovery can demonstrate the positive effects of the process and demonstrate to your partner the benefits of joining you in it. Both the research and our clinical experience have shown that in at least half of the cases in which the injured partner started out working alone toward recovery, hope for the relationship was renewed and the partner who had the affair made new efforts to participate.

3. **Do the end-of-chapter exercises by yourself.** Some are designed for you as an individual; others will be for you as a couple. In many cases you can do the couple exercises if you just change them a bit; we'll help you do that.

EXERCISES

The goal of the exercises at the end of each chapter is to help you take what you've been reading and apply it to your own situation. You'll move closer to recovery as you bring these ideas to life in your own relationship.

Some exercises will suggest that you write things down. We recommend that you create a notebook or use an electronic device where you keep your responses, no matter how brief or how detailed. If you're work-ing with your partner, it might be good for each of you to have a separate record of your responses. For the exercise that follows for this chapter, we recommend that even if you and your partner are working through the book together, you do it separately and not share your responses with each other for now. Take some time by yourself to look at what's happen-ing for *you* right now.

At times later in the book, we'll suggest you go back and see how things have changed during this journey, so writing down your responses can help you see your progress. Take whatever time you need for each exercise. Give yourself the gift of time to focus and understand and to plan for the future.

EXERCISE 1.1 Understanding Your Reactions to What's Happened

Before you can change something, you need to be aware of what's hap-pening. For now, we want to make sure you know what's happening to you individually. Later we'll ask you to try to understand your partner and the affair.

Look again at the lists of common reactions following discovery of an affair described on pages 13–16 in this chapter—including common thoughts, feelings, and behaviors. Use those descriptions to help clarify what your own experiences have been.

Thoughts, Assumptions, and Boundaries

Affairs not only make you feel bad; they also tear away some of your core beliefs about your partner, your relationship, and maybe even yourself. *List your major beliefs or views about your partner, your relationship, or yourself that have been damaged or have changed as a result of the affair. What boundaries have been crossed?* For example:

> "What's most upsetting to me is that I thought you were the one per-son in my life I could count on to care for me, and now I can't." Or "It seemed so clear to me that we wouldn't behave that way with other people; how can you say it's no big deal and I'm overreacting?" Or "I always thought I was weak and couldn't make it on my own. But since dealing with this, I actually think I'm stronger than I realized."

Feelings

What are the main feelings you're having now and since the affair was revealed? Are you angry, sad, or frightened? Confused or numb? Relieved at having it in the open? Have you had any good feelings as you've talked with your partner—warm, close, reassured, or some other feelings?

List your major feelings and try to link them to what you're thinking at the time or to what's just happened. For example:

> "I get furious when you refuse to talk to me about what happened." Or "I get really frustrated when you ask me the same questions night after night." Or "Whenever we work through really painful discussions together, I feel more hopeful."

Behaviors

When you and your partner are this upset, you might behave in ways that aren't typical for you. This is understandable, given the situation, but if you continue behaving this way for long, things probably won't get better or will even get worse. *List the major ways that you've started behaving differently as an individual that might get in the way of recovery or are making things worse.* For example:

> "I've been saying all kinds of cruel things to my partner, but sometimes that makes me feel worse about myself." Or "I'm withdrawing even though I know we have to talk." Or "I'm now checking on my partner constantly—where they are, what they're doing, questioning them about their whereabouts many times a day."

You might also be acting in some new ways that you feel good about. List those too. For example:

> "I'm standing up for myself now, and that feels good." Or "I'm being totally honest now. If that creates conflict between us, then we'll just have to deal with that. But I like the new, honest part of me."

2

How Do We Get Through the Day?

Allison first suspected Seth's affair when a friend said she'd seen him having "an intimate dinner" with another woman when Allison was out of town. Years earlier, Seth had been involved in a brief affair, but the couple had put it behind them and never really discussed it after the first couple of weeks. This time, Allison insisted that Seth move out.

At first, Seth and Allison continued to see each other after work to try to sort through what had happened. Allison insisted on knowing every detail of the affair, and initially Seth answered most of her questions. But when she demanded to know the other woman's name and address, Seth refused and stopped communicating with Allison for several weeks. When they finally talked again, Allison asked him to move back home so they could work things out. Seth agreed to do whatever he could to work on their relationship, but only on the condition that they wouldn't discuss his affair anymore.

Having a break from the heated arguments that arose whenever they discussed Seth's affair was a relief. But soon Allison found herself still wondering about the affair and questioning Seth's honesty. She felt uncomfortable when he tried to kiss her or initiate lovemaking, and Seth accused her of not really wanting to get close again. Before they knew it, they were hardly speaking. Neither one wanted a divorce, but it felt as if the gap between them was widening every day.

Right after an affair comes to light, life feels unsafe. Most couples describe their relationship as chaotic. Now that all the "givens" have been destroyed and the rules violated, they have no idea how to interact just to get through the day. How should you and your partner try to deal with what's happening in your relationship? How do you communicate without letting your feelings get out of control? What should you talk about? How do you manage routine activities like preparing meals, taking care of the children, or paying bills? How affectionate does either of you feel toward the other, and what should you do if you differ in this area? *Most important, how do you and your partner avoid making things worse?*

Couples usually react in one of three ways, and often they try various approaches because nothing seems to work:

1. Some couples try to go on as if nothing has happened.
2. Other couples frantically try to get closer—for example, spending most of their time together or making love more often in an attempt to save their relationship.
3. Still other couples try to get some distance from each other, which can reduce unproductive conflict but inadvertently deepen mistrust.

Here's the advice we often give couples trying to deal with the immediate aftermath of an affair:

✍ For now, just focus on trying not to make things worse.

There's not a lot of *recovery* that's likely to happen right now. But the chances of your recovering down the road could be strongly affected by decisions you make about how to deal with things over the next month or two. Not making things worse is what this chapter and the next two are all about.

Setting healthy boundaries is probably the most important way to avoid making things worse. You're going to need boundaries between your partner and you, between you two and the outside affair person, and between you two and other people who may or may not need to be told about the affair.

The boundaries you'll need first, just to get through each day, are the ones between you and your partner, so these are discussed here. But if you find that too many conversations quickly spiral out of control, turn to Chapter 3 now for specific communication skills and strategies. Or if the involved partner has not yet ended the affair, you may want to skip ahead and read the relevant portion of Chapter 4 before reading the rest of this chapter.

Setting Boundaries between You and Your Partner

"We just can't get away from it," Zuri complained. "It's the same thing every night. Question after question after question. Jaden never lets up. It feels like an inquisition, and I can't take it anymore. I know what I did was wrong, and I've sworn to Jaden and myself not to lie anymore. But our talks aren't making things better; they're making things worse. And if I say, 'Enough!' and want to stop for the night, he gets furious."

Should We Talk About the Affair?

Most couples find it impossible *not* to talk about the affair. Talking about the affair is one way of communicating hurt and trying to reestablish security: "How could you do this? Isn't our relationship important to you anymore?" The trouble is, you and your partner may not agree about whether or how to talk about the affair or how much to discuss or reveal. It's important to understand what you do need to talk about and how to set boundaries that help you to have these discussions without making things worse. Exercise 2.1 at the end of this chapter can help you accomplish this.

As difficult as it can be for people like Zuri, talking about the affair is probably the only way of coming to a full understanding of how the affair came about and how to prevent it from happening again. However, not all couples do talk about a partner's affair—at least not initially. Talking about an affair can be painful and frightening. Sometimes a person is reluctant to discuss their affair because the partner's pain becomes even more evident at those times. It can be particularly challenging when one person wants to discuss the affair and the other one doesn't. *Not discussing the affair may avoid some discomfort in the short run but is likely to result in more difficulties in the long run.*

When Zuri disclosed her affair to Jaden, he said he was hurt but would try to understand. At first he asked that they both put the affair out of their minds, but months later his attitude seemed to change. He wanted to know everything. How did Zuri's lover kiss? Exactly what did they do sexually? The more vivid the images became, the more haunting they were, and soon Jaden could think of nothing else. Zuri and Jaden struggled to distinguish between discussions they needed to have to reestablish emotional security and discussions they needed to avoid because they would likely make recovery more difficult.

What Do We Talk About and Not Talk About?

When a couple first begins to talk about one partner's affair, three overriding questions are important to consider:

- What happened?
- Why did you do it?
- Where does this leave us?

WHAT HAPPENED?

In discussing "what happened," couples need to reach a common understanding about the basic events of the affair. Affairs involve crossing boundaries that are vital for a couple's well-being. What kinds of boundaries have been violated during this affair? In the box on the facing page we've listed some common questions that couples usually need to address after a partner's infidelity. You need to know when the affair began, how long it lasted, and when and how it ended. For example, a one-time sexual encounter in unusual circumstances may have a different meaning and different effects on a relationship than a six-month affair with a close friend of the couple. Zuri's affair was a weeklong "fling" that included one instance of sexual intimacy during Jaden's two-month business trip in Europe. Although it was Zuri's guilt that caused her to disclose her infidelity to her husband, in

What Happened?

- When did the affair begin? Is this person someone you've known for a while? When did the relationship first become flirtatious, and when did it become sexual (if it was sexual)?

- Who initiated the affair? Did either one of you try to stop it and, if so, how?

- Is the other person married or in a committed relationship? Does that person's partner know? If not, do you or the affair person intend to tell the other partner?

- Exactly what kinds of boundaries were crossed during the affair?

- When and where did you get together? How many times did you and the other person engage in sexual activity, if at all?

- How much emotional involvement was there? How frequently did you and the outside person talk with or write to each other? What else did you do together?

- What kinds of contraception or protection against sexually transmitted infections (STIs) were used? Did you ever not use protection? Have you or the other person been tested for STIs?

- How much money was spent on the affair? What do you intend to do with any gifts or other mementos from the affair?

- Has the affair ended? If so, when and by whom? If the affair has ended, is this just for now or permanently?

- What contact have you had with the outside person since then? What steps, if any, have you taken to ensure that no further contact takes place? What are your plans if the outside person contacts you?

- Who else knows about the affair? What do others know, and how did they find out?

- Are there any other consequences we need to consider, such as complications at work or legal problems? Could the outside person or their partner make our lives more difficult if they wanted to?

her mind it *could* be put behind them because it was such a fleeting event in their lives and was not an ongoing threat to them. Jaden seemed to agree at first, but the emotional fallout turned out to be just as devastating as if it had gone on for months. The intensity and duration of an affair are important to get out in the open because these factors could have significant implications for moving forward.

You may also want and need to know something about the outside affair person and the nature of the affair so you can move forward. What was the outside person's role in initiating or maintaining the affair? Was the affair mostly emotional or sexual? Some research suggests that women sometimes find emotional involvement of their partners with someone else particularly threatening, whereas men often react more strongly to their partners' sexual involvement with someone else. However, no matter your gender, other research suggests that all people feel threatened when they think that their most intimate, important relationships are in danger.

It's only natural to want to understand the "magnitude and type of threat" from an outside person, and that's why if you're the injured party, you probably can't help focusing on what your partner and the affair person actually did together. What happened already is likely extremely painful, but is there the risk of its happening again or your relationship actually ending? For some people, assessing the potential social threat from others becoming involved is also important. Learning of a partner's affair is shocking enough. The last thing you need on top of that is to worry about who knows what and who is talking about you behind your back or to be blindsided by an outsider's comments.

Of course, there may also be actual physical threats that need to be considered. Foremost among these is the risk of a sexually transmitted infection (STI). If unprotected sex occurred even once, both of you should be evaluated medically for risks or indications of an STI. Separate from issues of risk for disease are threats of physical violence. We've worked with couples in situations where the outside affair person reacted to the unwanted ending of an affair by becoming physically aggressive toward either the involved or injured partner. On occasion, the outside person's own partner has become physically aggressive toward the involved partner or tried to ruin their reputation by making things public. We're not proposing undue alarm, but we do suggest a candid and realistic discussion of potential physical aggression or other forms of retaliation from anyone involved in the affair, either directly or indirectly.

What couples should avoid discussing are the intimate details of the affair—especially in terms of specific sexual behaviors. Jaden's insistence that Zuri disclose everything she and her affair partner did in bed together didn't bring him emotional security; it didn't make him feel better about Zuri, himself, or their marriage, and it didn't provide information that led to understanding or how to move forward. Instead, it made it even harder for Jaden to replace images of the affair in his mind with more helpful visions of times when he and Zuri had been at their best together, or of how they could reach that state again.

Of course, knowing what matters need to be discussed isn't always enough to ensure productive conversations. Like Zuri and Jaden, you might find that you and your partner end up in escalating arguments or prolonged withdrawals that leave you both with mounting frustration and resentment. If that's the case, turn to Chapter 3, where we offer guidelines for talking about feelings productively—and for listening well too.

WHY DID YOU DO IT?

Gaining a full understanding of how the affair came about is critical to regaining a sense of security and making good decisions about how to move on. So you may be surprised to see that the box below about why the affair happened contains so few items. This isn't because we consider this question unimportant or expect it to be "in the background" following the initial discovery or disclosure of an affair. It's often the most consuming question that injured partners have. However, prolonged, detailed

Why Did You Do It?

- Why do you think the affair happened?
- What were you thinking about me and our family?
- Why didn't you tell me? (Or why did you wait to tell me?)

discussions about why the affair occurred aren't likely to be very productive or satisfying at this time; they'll become central later on. One reason
is that the involved partner often doesn't really *know* why. Later in the
recovery process we've heard, "I must have been crazy. What on earth was
I thinking?" or "The more I've looked at things, the more I realize that
most of my initial beliefs about why I had the affair were wrong." Pushing
for conclusive answers now will likely produce only inaccurate or incomplete explanations, which can get in the way of looking more closely at the
bigger picture later on.

Another reason that probing for "Why?" is often unproductive is that
your partner knows that no explanation is likely to reassure you and therefore doesn't want to talk about it. Your partner may also sincerely want
to avoid causing you further pain by discussing their own relationship
unhappiness or disappointments. Some people who have an affair also
feel such deep shame and self-loathing afterward that persistent questions
about "why" can begin to feel intolerable.

So, rather than suggesting that you avoid the "why" questions entirely,
we advise you for now to avoid spending endless hours going over the same
questions. Some couples literally exhaust themselves staying up talking
night after night and still feel they're getting nowhere. Part II of this book
is devoted to examining how the affair came about; try to be patient and
wait until you've read through Part I before pushing for full answers to
these questions.

WHERE DOES THIS LEAVE US?

Where the affair will leave you in the long run is probably still uncertain,
but there are some intermediate issues you may need to resolve in the short
term. Common questions addressing these concerns are listed in the box
on the facing page. Some of these—for example, how to deal with daily
family and household responsibilities and how to express emotional or
physical closeness—need to be addressed early on, though you need to
realize that the answers are likely to change over time. Others—such as
considering separation or divorce—are better dealt with later unless one
of you has already taken steps in this direction. In short, try to distinguish between immediate decisions that need to be made *now* and those
for which you'll be better informed *later,* after you've taken time to work

Where Does This Leave Us?

- What about us? Should we continue to live together for now?

- How do we make sure that we talk about the things that need to be talked about?

- How do we deal with the basic tasks of managing our relationship and our household?

- What acts of caring feel okay right now—for example, calling or texting during the day just to stay connected or having our morning coffee together?

- What other expressions of intimacy do we want? Are hugs or kisses okay? What about making love together?

- What do you think it would take for us to get through this just for now? What commitments are either of us ready to make about our relationship in the short term?

- Do you already know what you want in the long run? If so, how did you reach that decision, and how certain are you that your feelings won't change?

- Have you considered divorce, contacted an attorney, or set up a separate bank account? Can we agree to suspend any steps toward divorce until after we've tried to work through things together?

through the step-by-step process of exploring how the affair occurred and how to move on as outlined in Parts II and III of this book.

Among the more important issues you might be debating is whether to continue living together. ***In general, we usually advise couples not to separate during the initial stages of dealing with an affair unless they absolutely can't remain together for the time being.*** Reestablishing a sense of security in your relationship is often vital to recovery, and separation can make this more difficult. In addition, you and your partner will need to discuss many issues to move on successfully, and separating before you do so can make it more difficult to talk about them later. If you have children, a separation may not be in their best interest. Separating sometimes encourages the outside affair person to pursue the involved partner even more aggressively, which usually deepens the wounds rather than healing them. Finally, separating may be a step toward a public announcement of the affair, which can lead to other complications, discussed in Chapter 4.

With that said, however, under certain circumstances it may be a good idea to separate. We've listed the most important of those situations in the box below.

Related to the issue of a separation, you each need to know whether the other has taken any steps to pursue a divorce. *Thoughts* about divorce aren't uncommon at times like this. But if either partner has consulted an attorney or has recently set up separate financial accounts, it's important that the other partner be aware of what's happening. Part of the damage from an affair is the secrecy and deceit; don't make things worse by taking other significant actions that your partner doesn't know about. The goal at this point isn't to "win." Rather, the goal is to ensure that whatever long-term decisions you reach, you're both able to move on with dignity and without hurting one another or others you care about.

Each of you should tell the other what you want and need in terms of the relationship for now. That doesn't necessarily mean deciding what you want to do about your relationship in the long run. By and large, we think that most couples often aren't prepared to make definite long-term decisions because they don't yet have all the information they need and their emotions are overwhelming. Instead, we're talking here about short-term

When a Separation Following an Affair Is a Good Decision

- *When one of you is absolutely certain of your decision to pursue a divorce.* It may be easier to separate now and move ahead with the divorce process, but be cautious. What seems certain now may not seem as clear just a few weeks ahead.

- *When you can't avoid repeated intense and verbally aggressive arguments* (even using the strategies in Chapter 3). Separating for now may be your last resort for not making things worse.

- *When the emotional turmoil in your relationship is contributing to physical aggression*—pushing, restraining, slapping, or worse.

decisions concerning the relationship. Do you each want to consider the possibility of making it work? Are you each prepared to commit to a process of examining how the affair came about and what it means for you both in the long run? Can you enter this process together?

How Can We Start to Return to Normal or Create a "New Normal"?

For Madison and Chase, everything felt awkward after Chase confessed his affair. Madison described it as "walking on broken glass" because they had to treat each other so gingerly. They knew they couldn't continue in their relationship like this, but they weren't sure how to take even the first steps toward getting back on track.

Once you decide whether you're going to continue living together, you may need to discuss how to handle matters that you no longer deal with automatically. Among them are tasks that just keep the relationship or family moving along. You need to look at what daily tasks have been disrupted by the affair and decide how they'll be carried out now. Will you divide up household responsibilities as you did before? Can you still do any of these tasks jointly? Can you handle them individually when they benefit both of you? If not, can you agree on a new system for getting things done so that neither one of you is hurt further and your relationship doesn't experience more damage? Exercise 2.2 will help you answer these questions.

Then there are the acts of caring that for now feel awkward. Maybe you used to call or text each other during the day just to reconnect. Or you may have exchanged small gestures, such as offering to get each other something from the kitchen before bedtime. Retreating into sustained silence for days or weeks on end can eat away at the foundation of your relationship. By contrast, finding a way to continue some of the previous acts of caring says, "I know things aren't resolved, and I know there's still hurt and tension between us. But I'm doing this to let you know that I still care, and I'm not giving up yet." When couples aren't able to engage in "joint" activities such as playing games together or going out to dinner where conversation is expected, we encourage "parallel" activities that allow you to be together without requiring a lot of interaction—perhaps

watching a movie together or attending a sporting event or theater pro-
duction together. You need to strike a balance here. Make an effort to be
thoughtful and considerate, but also recognize that you may not be comfortable right now with some of the ways you've shown love or affection in
the past.

Finally, deciding how to handle intimate aspects of your relationship,
including both sex and physical affection, can be particularly difficult. Are
you each comfortable with gentle touches? What about hugs or kisses? Are
you ready to sleep together? If you've stopped making love, are you ready
to become sexually intimate again? We've seen people differ tremendously
in their preferences along these lines. For some couples, making love following an affair can be an important way of reconnecting and comforting
one another, while still acknowledging that parts of the relationship feel
uncertain. For other couples, even gentle touches can feel uncomfortable.
We don't advocate any one way of dealing with this area over another.
What's important is that you and your partner discuss this in ways that
aren't demanding or hostile.

You may both decide to try to return to some of your well-established
ways of interacting with each other. However, some of those previous ways
of interacting may not work, particularly if they make you feel too vulnerable, and you may need to create new patterns or a "new normal" for
now. Those decisions likely will depend on how each of you is doing right
now and what types of boundaries were crossed in the affair. If the affair
included lots of sexual activity, reengaging sexually with your partner
might not work at present; if there was a great deal of emotional closeness
in the affair, you might not want to open up and be vulnerable with your
partner right now.

Decisions you make in the short run won't prevent you from reaching
different decisions down the road. Moreover, you should anticipate fluc-
tuations in how either one of you feels about emotional or sexual intimacy,
particularly the injured partner. What feels comfortable and soothing
today may feel awkward or even traumatic tomorrow, and vice versa. Probably the best way to find out what your partner wants is to ask. Too often
people try to read each other's body language and misinterpret what the
other person wants. Such misunderstandings can escalate quickly when
they're not checked with direct questions: "When I touched you last night,
you pulled back from me. I'm wondering what you were feeling then?"

Why Do Things Sometimes Suddenly Fall Apart? Coping with Flashbacks

If setting boundaries is the most important way to avoid making things worse, learning to cope with flashbacks comes in a close second. When you and your partner seem to be doing better but then things suddenly fall apart, it's easy to feel as if you've erased everything you gained—and then some.

> Jake and Megan were driving along the highway on their way to a nearby resort for the weekend. They felt good about the progress they'd made toward recovering from Megan's affair a few months ago, and both had really looked forward to this getaway together. Suddenly Jake stopped talking, and when Megan turned toward him, she noticed he was gripping the wheel tightly and his expression was grim. What had she said that had upset him? When she asked him what was wrong, Jake said they'd just driven by a motel of the same chain where Megan and the outside person involved in the affair had sometimes gone in their hometown. Seeing another motel of the same name had made Jake feel sick to his stomach all over again.
>
> Megan instantly plunged into despair. She feared they would never recover, no matter what she did. She could never see these mood swings coming. Why did he have to bring up her affair, at this of all times, and ruin their weekend? Why couldn't he just agree to move on?

Jake and Megan's struggles with reminders of her affair demonstrate an inevitable part of the recovery process. Driving by a motel of a similar name, seeing a car of the model owned by the outside person, or hearing a text message arrive on your partner's phone can stir up memories of those deeply painful, traumatic feelings that accompanied the discovery of a partner's affair. And besides the personally relevant details that trigger flashbacks, TV, newspapers, and movies are filled with references to infidelity. Reexperiencing the affair, even when both partners are convinced that the affair has ended, often occurs at unpredictable times and is nearly always deeply distressing for both.

We're going to emphasize here the kinds of acutely distressing flashbacks frequently experienced by injured partners. But involved partners can also struggle with memories that stir up guilt, shame, or even sometimes feelings for the outside person, and the guidelines offered on the next few pages may be helpful for dealing with these as well.

How Can I Recognize When I'm Having a Flashback?

In the strictest sense, *flashback* refers to a reexperiencing of a traumatic incident with the same emotional, cognitive, and physiological reactions felt at the time the trauma occurred. But if you think of flashbacks as occurring along a continuum, with true reexperiencing at one end and experiences more like upsetting memories at the other, flashbacks related to affairs often fall somewhere in the middle. The memories are painful enough to disrupt your thoughts and feelings, but typically you're fully aware that the trigger is distinct from the event itself. Flashbacks at any level involve painful feelings, memories, and images from the past. Because they occur suddenly and unexpectedly, they typically feel unpredictable and beyond your control.

Flashbacks usually are very upsetting to both partners. But they can become even more distressing when misunderstood or mismanaged. Often, the involved partner concludes that the injured partner is experiencing the flashback intentionally, unwilling to let go, or using the flashback experience to punish them. The injured person can feel frightened, overwhelmed, and hopeless about ever getting over it. Therefore, unless you and your partner develop an effective way of recognizing and responding to flashbacks, they can disrupt your progress and ultimately block your recovery. Guidelines for coping with flashbacks are summarized in the box on the facing page. Exercise 2.3 at the end of this chapter will help you and your partner use these guidelines in developing specific strategies for dealing with flashbacks.

If you're having flashbacks, you need to decide on when and how to share these. Following the initial discovery of an affair, you'll probably experience many reminders that trigger sadness, hurt, fear, or anger. However, asking your partner to discuss with you *every* memory you have of the affair, or every reexperiencing no matter what the level of intensity, can eventually wear your partner down. So try to evaluate the importance of discussing your flashback in any given situation. If your memory or flashback is highly distressing to you and you need support, if it's interfering with your ability to interact constructively with your partner, or if your

Guidelines for Coping with Flashbacks

- If you recognize that you're responding to your partner in a worried or angry manner, step back and evaluate the situation and your reaction.

- If you decide that your reaction is realistic given the immediate circumstances, express your feelings to your partner and work to find a more acceptable solution. For example: *"When you're an hour late getting home from work and haven't called, it makes me worry about where you are and what you're doing—just like I used to worry right after your affair. Let's discuss how to handle occasions when you get delayed unexpectedly."*

- If you decide that your reaction is most likely a reaction to a memory of the affair, let your partner know what is happening by describing your feelings and linking them to the memory that has been triggered. For example: *"Driving by that motel just triggered memories of your affair, and I feel hurt and frightened all over again."*

- Try to distinguish among the different feelings you're having and how aroused you're becoming physically. For example: *"When your phone just buzzed while we were sleeping, I flashed back to those texts you would get late at night during your affair. My heart is pounding, and it feels just as intense as it did back then."*

- Be specific about what would be most helpful at this moment in dealing with these feelings. Do you simply want your partner to acknowledge your feelings? Do you want to be held or reassured, or given time and space to be by yourself? For example: *"I've been feeling more alone and distant from you today. I really need you to be with me and just hold me for a while."*

- Work with your partner to reduce the likelihood of these triggers in the future. For example: *"Watching movies together used to be fun, but right now I really need us to avoid movies about romance, infidelity, or other reminders of your affair. How can we manage that?"*

- Balance discussions with your partner about flashbacks with efforts to deal with these experiences on your own to avoid overwhelming your relationship or wearing down your partner with these difficult interactions.

partner asks about your feelings during a flashback, you should probably discuss it. But sometimes it will be important for you to try to cope with these experiences on your own. In balancing your efforts to cope with flashbacks as a couple versus dealing with them on your own, use some of the self-care strategies described in Chapter 5.

How Should I Respond to My Partner's Flashbacks?

Involved partners need to know how to respond to their injured partner's flashbacks without making things worse. If you think your partner may be experiencing a flashback or other emotional reaction to memories of your affair, ask if this is so and invite your partner to share these feelings with you. Your partner may prefer not to talk with you about it. If so, try to accept that decision for now. More likely, your partner will interpret your offer as your willingness to listen in an effort to offer support or understanding. Use the guidelines for effective listening offered in Chapter 3. Describe specifically what you're observing in your partner without attacking and ask your partner to clarify what they're feeling: "You seem quiet all of a sudden, and you look pretty tense. Do you want to talk about what's going on?"

Try to help your partner identify the trigger (or triggers) for what they're currently feeling. What brought on the flashback? Is it something you've said or done without realizing it? Was it some other trigger in the environment? Was it something inside your partner—such as worrying about not measuring up to the outside person or suddenly seeing an image of the other person? When your partner identifies the trigger, try to avoid becoming defensive. For example, if your partner describes experiencing a flashback when you get a text message at night, that doesn't mean your partner believes you're having an affair all over again. You don't need to defend yourself or insist that your partner stop having such thoughts. Instead you can respond, "I'm sorry this happened to you. I know it feels terrible. Let's try to get through it together." Try to listen and be caring; it doesn't mean you've just done something wrong.

In addition to clarifying the particular trigger at the moment, consider talking about the things that tend to trigger such intense feelings for each of you. Identifying these triggers can help both of you recognize high-risk situations. In some cases, you can rearrange things to avoid likely triggers—for example, avoid staying late at work alone. Some triggers can't always be avoided, but recognizing triggers in advance can help you reduce their occurrence and manage their impact more effectively.

What Can I Do to Help Right Now?

Inviting your injured partner to describe what they want from you in this moment can help the two of you work together to deal with these difficult experiences. Your partner's desires may change across different situations. Sometimes they may simply want to be held or reassured of your love and that you'll be there. Other times they may want to express their feelings or discuss how to avoid certain triggers in the future. On other occasions, your partner might want time and space to deal with the flashback on their own.

Anticipate that at times your partner may not be sure what they want or may say one thing at first and feel differently later. So be patient and try to remain flexible. If your partner initially asks to be left alone, check back again later and see if their feelings have changed and they now prefer to have you nearby. Most important is that you approach these flashbacks as a couple. First clarify whether your partner is having some type of flashback experience so there are no misunderstandings; then talk about what your partner needs and what you can do right now to be helpful.

What Should We Expect Regarding These Setbacks?

For now, you should probably anticipate that flashbacks at various levels will continue. And just when these experiences seem to be behind you, they'll pop up again in ways that may feel discouraging. But flashbacks don't mean that you're back to square one, that your partner isn't trying, or the situation is hopeless. They're a typical part of the recovery process. In our experience, flashbacks gradually diminish in frequency, intensity, and their impact on both partners. You can facilitate this process by staying hopeful, working together, and using the guidelines outlined here.

The next chapter describes strategies for expressing and responding to each other's feelings, making decisions together, and lowering the temperature during heated discussions. Because so many of these skills and strategies are useful in dealing with the matters discussed in this chapter, many people find it helpful to read Chapters 2 and 3 together to consider how to integrate skills from Chapter 3 into their Chapter 2 work. You can always come back to the Chapter 2 exercises after learning more about effective communication strategies described in Chapter 3.

EXERCISES

The following exercises are designed to help you and your partner deal with challenges in interacting. It's best for the two of you to do them together, but you can benefit from doing them separately too, if needed.

■ *If you're working with your partner:* First read through the exercises separately and write down your individual responses. Then schedule a time to exchange and discuss your responses. Limit any discussion to 30 minutes even if that means discussing only one question or part of a question—better to do that effectively than to rush through the questions or spend too much time and end up tired, discouraged, or hurt. You're more likely to come back and try again if you can keep your discussions constructive.

■ *If you're working through this book separately or alone:* Read through the exercises on your own and write down your individual responses. Consider whether your partner might be willing to sit down with you and talk about the issues addressed. If so, agree on a time when you both have 15–30 minutes to begin considering these issues one at a time. The more constructive you can make these initial discussions, the more likely your partner may be to engage in more difficult discussions down the road. Use the exercises to decide how *you* would like to interact with your partner. Focus on your own behaviors. Regardless of where you two end up, you're likely to feel better about yourself if you can look back and know that you managed your own behaviors as well as possible.

EXERCISE 2.1 Talking About the Affair

What to Talk About

Your discussions are likely to go better if you can limit the number of questions you present to your partner at this time and make your questions as specific as possible. *List the top five questions you'd most like to talk with your partner about at this time.* Try to focus on information you need to have now to get through the next few weeks. For example:

> "When did the affair begin? What contact do you still have with the outside person?"

> "Was there ever a time when you didn't use protection against a sexually transmitted infection?"

> "Have you already decided to end our relationship?"

Avoid the "why" questions as much as possible for now. We'll get to these important questions at a later time. To keep the discussion from being one-sided, you might consider asking your partner to list the top few questions that they would like to ask you.

When and Where to Talk About It

Your discussion will probably go better if you and your partner agree on when, where, and for how long to have your first few discussions. *Write down your proposal for when and where to have your initial discussions with your partner about the affair. Share this proposal with your partner and try to reach a specific agreement. If your partner doesn't agree with your initial proposal, explore other possibilities.* For example:

> "Let's sit down for 30 minutes Tuesday evening in the living room after the children go to bed to begin discussing my top five questions. During that time, we agree not to get distracted by our phones or work or TV. After 30 minutes, regardless of where we are, we'll stop for the night and continue another time."

EXERCISE 2.2 Deciding How to Interact for Now

Many areas of the relationship, from handling chores to physical intimacy, may feel confusing or uncertain to you or your partner right now. It's important to work toward decisions that specify what each of you will do or not do and what the trial period will be, such as the next few days or the next few weeks.

If you and your partner are unable to reach tentative decisions in the areas emphasized below, you may want to draw on the specific guidelines for decision making discussed in Chapter 3.

Managing Basic Tasks

You and your partner probably need to reach decisions about a variety of chores. *List the top five tasks or areas of responsibility that you and your partner will need to decide how to handle to get through the next week or two. For each of these, state what the task or concern is and propose some possible solutions.* For example:

> "We need to decide how to handle the kids' activities after school. I suggest that we continue the same transportation plans we've used in the past. I'd like us both to continue to attend their events and sit together, but without the need to talk with each other if we don't feel like it."

Or

> "I'd like you to continue to pay the bills, but I'd like a brief update every week on what's been paid out and what our bank balance is so I can be better informed about our finances."

Engaging in Acts of Caring

In the past, you and your partner may have exchanged simple acts of caring that now feel uncertain or awkward—for example, calling or texting just to stay connected, going for a walk together, or making the other person a snack. If it feels appropriate, *list four or five ways that you'd like you and your partner to engage in simple acts of caring over the next few weeks. As you list these, try to include one or two behaviors in each of these categories:*

- *Unilateral: Things either of you can do on your own for the other.* For example:

  > "I'd like you to help with our kids' daycare afternoon pickups this week" or "I'd like you to continue to make coffee for me in the morning."

- *Parallel: Things you do together but that don't require much interaction.* For example:

  > "I'd like us to watch a movie together."

■ *Joint: Things that you do together that involve direct interaction.* For example:

> "I'd like to go to dinner with you and just enjoy ourselves, with no discussion of what happened. I need some time together that feels relaxed and safe."

Dealing with Your Physical and Sexual Relationship

You and your partner need to decide how you're going to deal with your physical relationship over the next few weeks. Your feelings about this may change over time, so it will be important to have a strategy for how to check back with each other on this occasionally. Because the two of you may have different preferences concerning your level of affectionate and sexual involvement right now, the guideline we encourage is to limit these exchanges to the safest level needed by either partner. *List the level of physical or sexual involvement that you would like to have with your partner over the next week or two. Describe who you'd like to be responsible for initiating these interactions and how you'd like to handle it if either one of you becomes uncomfortable during these times.* For example:

> "Sometimes I need us to make love because it feels reassuring to me. Other times I'm not comfortable with you even touching me. I'd like for either one of us to be able to give the other a simple hug outside of the bedroom. But, for now, to feel safe I want to be the one to initiate anything more than that—including making love or even kissing. If we're beginning to become more intimate and it starts to feel uncomfortable for either one of us, I want either of us to be able to say so and for us to stop what we're doing without any explanation required and without either of us getting angry toward the other."

EXERCISE 2.3 Coping with Flashbacks

Because flashbacks are so common following an affair and can interfere with recovery, it's important for you and your partner to try to understand how they come about and develop plans for coping with them.

Recognizing a Flashback

Try to recall different times when you suddenly found yourself thinking about the affair at an unexpected time or place. What thoughts and feelings were you having? Or try to recall times when you became aware that your partner was experiencing a flashback linked to the affair. What did your partner do or say? What did you observe on your own? *Describe as many signs or aspects of your own or your partner's flashback experiences as you can identify.*

Identifying Triggers

Try to identify as many triggers as possible for these flashback experiences. Where were you, and where was your partner? What was each of you doing? What was happening before and at the time of the flashback? The more specifically you can identify triggers of flashbacks, the more you and your partner may be able to minimize their happening. If you were with your partner and noticed a sudden change in their mood that seemed unrelated to what was happening between the two of you, can you recall what else was going on at the time? *Describe as many triggers for your own or your partner's flashback experiences as you can identify.*

Coping with Flashbacks

Try to develop as many ways of coping with flashbacks as you can. Some of these should be for you together as a couple; others should be for the person experiencing the flashback to cope with on their own.

Explore strategies for you and your partner to cope with flashbacks together. For example, how can you let your partner know if you're experiencing a flashback? Or if your partner's mood or behaviors suddenly change in ways that you believe may be linked to a flashback, how can you ask about it in a way that reflects your concern and willingness to help? Once you're both aware that one of you is experiencing a flashback, what steps can you take to reduce the duration or impact of this experience? For example, if the person experiencing the flashback initially wants separate time and space alone, should the other partner still check back later to see whether this need has changed to a wish for closeness and reassurance?

Similarly, identify ways for you to cope with flashbacks on your own. For example, does meditation or pursuing individual activities such as exercise shorten or decrease the intensity of the flashback? Or does engaging with others such as a family member or close friend help you gain a sense of calm? Remind yourself that these flashbacks don't mean that you'll never recover. For each of these strategies for coping with flash-backs, identify any assistance you may need from your partner, such as providing an opportunity to be by yourself or help in watching the children while you engage with others. If you have difficulty thinking of strategies for coping with flashback experiences on your own, turn to Chapter 5 for suggestions on how to care for yourself better.

3

How Do We Talk with Each Other?

When Will discovered Courtney's affair, what happened next followed a familiar pattern: Will threatened divorce, and Courtney broke off her brief affair almost immediately. They argued constantly, and Will planned to move out. When he was starting to pack his bags, they both realized they weren't ready to end their 10-year marriage. They pulled back from the brink and found ways to limit their verbal battles. For several weeks, they forced themselves to continue family meals, go to the kids' soccer games together, figure out who would drive the kids where, and so on.

It didn't take long, however, for Courtney and Will to become painfully aware of the emptiness in their relationship. They were sleeping in the same bed but not making love. When they tried to talk about the affair and their relationship, neither could seem to find the right words to be understood. When Will tried to explain to Courtney that he felt wounded at a depth he had never experienced before, and why at times he still froze when she touched him, he just ended up repeating how hurt he was. In response, Courtney kept saying that she understood and was sorry for what she had done.

But Will didn't feel understood, and Courtney didn't know what else to say. She knew Will was devastated, but repeating how sorry she was and that she understood seemed to have little impact. It hurt when she felt his pain, knowing she had caused it, *but Courtney also struggled with her own hurt. For several years she had tried to tell Will how shut out she felt from his life. She had no longer felt important to him, and this feeling had partly led to her looking for support and attention elsewhere. Still, there was just no way she could tell Will this—not after what she had done. Yet, until he understood, how could they really begin to rebuild their relationship?*

Eventually Will grew tired of trying to explain how he felt, and Courtney seemed tired of trying to understand.

Feeling understood by your partner is one of the most important parts of an intimate relationship. Most people enter into a long-term committed relationship because they feel special to each other—able to talk about deep feelings and disclose parts of themselves that they ordinarily wouldn't share with anyone else, or have a deep sense of understanding one another without needing to share verbally. Being able to share deep feelings, to have these feelings heard and understood, and to experience warm and tender caring form the very core of intimacy.

An affair shatters this foundation of intimacy, especially for the injured partner. The person you counted on the most to be faithful and to provide caring when life is difficult is no longer reliable. It no longer feels safe to express feelings that make you vulnerable, so much of your hurt may be expressed as anger or rage. Sometimes the shock and pain are so deep that you may go numb just to get through the day. At other times, the anger may combine with self-doubts to produce a deep depression. Anger and depression, or attack and withdrawal, may alternate in rapid or unpredictable ways. In the midst of this chaos, being able to express yourself clearly, in a way that can be heard and understood by your partner, is as difficult as it is vital.

If you're the involved partner, you may be struggling as well with your own feelings of hurt, anger, or shame, which may interfere with being able to listen and respond effectively to your partner's feelings.

In this chapter, we'll suggest some better ways of talking with your partner. We offer certain guidelines for expressing your feelings and for responding to your partner's feelings that can help your partner hear what you're trying to say and help you both *feel* heard and understood. When you both feel understood, you'll be better able to use the problem-solving skills described here too. And for the inevitable moments when discussions become too heated, we'll give guidelines for keeping things from escalating out of control.

Principles for Talking with Your Partner

When an affair has just become known, it's simply not reasonable to expect complete calm when you try to talk about it. It may help, however, to keep in mind three goals:

1. Keep the discussions balanced.
2. Keep conversations focused.
3. Prevent further damage.

Sticking to these key principles can be difficult, but here are specific tips that can help.

Maintaining Balance

One way to keep things from spinning out of control is to remember that the ultimate goal of your discussions is to find a way to move forward. As a general rule, we encourage involved partners to listen patiently and nondefensively to their injured partner's distress. But over time, intense negativity that is uninterrupted by anything positive can erode whatever hope there is for working together toward recovery. Instead, we suggest the injured partner also try to acknowledge what was once right with this relationship and what may be worth saving. Don't "rewrite" the history of your relationship to make it sound all bad, but also don't paint it as having been perfect until your partner ruined it with an affair.

Another way to keep the discussion balanced is to make sure both of you share your feelings and perspectives. To move forward, you need to come to a good understanding of *each other's* perspective, by stepping back from your own feelings and trying to listen to each other. That's easier said than done, we know. But try to put yourself in your partner's shoes and see things from their perspective.

Staying Focused

Keeping your discussions focused means not allowing the affair to intrude into almost every moment of every interaction. Some couples have found it helpful to agree on a time and place to discuss concerns related to the affair—for example, at night after the children have gone to bed. Others agree to a time limit on any one discussion—for example, 30 minutes. If you find it almost impossible to talk to one another without getting out of control, then writing down questions (just a few at a time) and providing written responses (more than one or two words!) can be a way of expressing concerns and sharing information in a more controlled way.

Keeping the affair from intruding is particularly critical at those times you set aside for comfort or pleasure together—for example, during special outings or during intimate times. *Work hard at preventing painful discussions during such times.* Another way to keep your discussions focused is to link whatever information you're seeking to specific steps or strategies for moving forward, such as "I want to know where you went out to dinner together, because for now, I just don't think I could handle going to the same places with you."

Preventing Further Damage

Avoiding making things worse may be the most important principle for discussing the affair. One way that damage occurs is from continuing arguments that escalate out of control and then saying or doing things that are deeply painful to one another. Recognize when your discussions start to get too heated and take a break until you can resume the discussion more constructively. We'll offer more specific guidance on this later.

Another way to prevent further damage is to clarify what you and your partner will discuss about the affair and in how much detail. One of the biggest problems couples may struggle with is how much explicit sexual detail the involved partner should reveal about the affair. *Our strong recommendation is that you not discuss these painful details with each other.* You need to know if your partner had intercourse with the other person, not specific details of who did what. Knowing more than that may create vivid mental images that will haunt you and make it even more difficult to move on. At the very least, hold off for now and see whether your desire for such information is as strong a few weeks or months down the road.

Talking About Feelings

How Can I Help My Partner Understand?

When you've tried to convey the same message repeatedly in different ways and it seems your partner still doesn't understand, you can't help believing that your partner needs to listen and respond more effectively. But it's also possible that your message isn't as clear as you think or that one or both of you are making assumptions that aren't accurate. Following these guidelines for expressing your feelings may help.

GENERAL GUIDELINES FOR DISCUSSING FEELINGS AS A COUPLE

■ *Work to understand and respond to your partner's feelings before expressing your own.* It's hard to really listen to the other person at the same time as you're thinking about what to say next, so try to focus on understanding what your partner is saying first rather than focusing on how you want to respond.

■ *Limit the feelings you're discussing to those that relate to a specific situation.* For example, if you're upset about something your partner said earlier in the day, don't allow the discussion to generalize to all the occasions when you've been upset over the past week.

■ *If you reach a point where it's clear that either of you isn't communicating well, take a break until you can come back and try again.* Talking about deep and difficult feelings well takes effort and practice. Doing it badly can inflict further damage and makes recovery more difficult. When you do take a break, be clear that you're not walking away from the discussion completely and let your partner know why you're taking the break (for example, "I'm feeling overwhelmed and need to cool down") and propose a time to pick the discussion back up.

■ *Be clear with each other about* why *you're communicating.* Are you just wanting to share thoughts and feelings, or are you trying to reach some sort of decision or solve a problem?

Sharing thoughts and feelings can help you feel connected, become more intimate, or get something off your chest. Conversations that focus on making decisions are more goal oriented and answer the question "What are we going to do?" Although both of these types of conversations are important—particularly for recovering from affairs—a common problem is that two partners can be pursuing different types of conversations at the same time. When this mismatch occurs, both partners are likely to feel frustrated.

> Kalisha continued to feel sad and confused months after learning of Jamal's affair. She was confident that his affair had ended and had seen Jamal's efforts to rebuild their relationship. But there were times when her deep hurt and her worries about whether they would survive as a couple washed over her. Jamal could tell when she was struggling and typically asked what he could do to reassure her or help her get past her feelings. Kalisha felt frustrated by his question. She just wanted him to understand that sometimes she still hurt and she still worried. Jamal felt equally frustrated. He had done everything she'd asked and more. He felt completely ineffective in helping Kalisha resolve her feelings. What else could he do?

Kalisha and Jamal's dilemma is common among couples struggling to recover from an affair. Sometimes the challenge isn't to "fix" feelings but simply to understand them. Kalisha learned that at those times it helped to begin the discussion by saying something like "Right now I just want you to understand what I'm feeling. I don't expect you to fix anything or do anything differently. But I've been feeling upset and alone, and I'd feel better if you at least understood what I'm experiencing."

The specific language you use isn't as important as being clear about whether you're trying to resolve something or just want to express your thoughts and feelings (see the box on the next page).

Sometimes Kalisha needed time to be by herself until she was able to get on top of her feelings and feel ready to interact with Jamal again. She learned to express that directly: "Jamal, right now I'm upset and need some

> When having a discussion about feelings:
>
> ■ Let your partner know that you're looking for understanding, not making a decision.
>
> ■ If there's a particular response you're hoping for—for example, being comforted or having separate time for yourself—tell your partner what you want.
>
> ■ If you're not sure whether your partner has started a discussion to share feelings or to resolve something or reach a decision, ask.

time for myself. It's not anything you've done or not done. I just need an evening by myself, and I hope you can understand that."

When Jamal wasn't clear on what type of conversation Kalisha wanted, he learned to ask: "I can tell you're upset, but I'm not sure what to do right now. Is this something we need to figure out how to deal with or do differently, or are you mostly just wanting me to listen to your feelings?" At other times he might say, "Kalisha, I know you're upset right now about the affair. Do you want to still try to be together right now, or would you prefer some time for yourself?"

SPECIFIC GUIDELINES FOR EXPRESSING YOUR FEELINGS

There are specific steps you can take to express your feelings in a way that may help your partner listen and understand. Following these guidelines may feel awkward at first, but if you adapt them to fit your personal speaking style, they'll begin to feel more natural. Choose one or two that seem easiest to start with, and gradually expand to include others.

■ *Speak for yourself, not for your partner.* One way to do this is to use an "I" statement that links your feelings to a specific situation or behavior. For example, "When you tell me just to forget it when I'm asking you about your affair, I feel unimportant to you." Or, "When you ask me where I've been but then don't believe me when I tell you, I feel frustrated and no longer feel like trying to answer your questions." Remember to focus on your own thoughts and feelings and allow your partner to speak for him- or herself.

■ *Express your feelings as your own subjective experience, not as absolute truths.* For example, instead of "You always ignore me" try "When you don't talk with me when you come in from work, I feel ignored."

■ *Focus on your feelings or emotions before moving on to thoughts or opinions.* Feelings are less likely to bring about a rebuttal than thoughts or opinions that accompany them.

■ *Be as specific as possible in describing your feelings.* The better able you are to describe specific feelings you're experiencing, the better your partner will be able to understand you. Consider, for example, the various ways to express both positive and negative feelings:

- o Positive feelings: Happy, close, secure, excited, calm, contented, fortunate, hopeful, inspired

- o Negative feelings: Hurt, discouraged, nervous, annoyed, weary, confused, lonely, ashamed

■ *When expressing negative feelings or concerns, also include any positive feelings you have.* Working toward a balanced expression of both positive and negative feelings may make it more likely that your negative feelings will be heard and that your partner will be able to respond to them in a more understanding way.

Following Avery's brief affair with one of her coworkers, Mark was uncomfortable with some of the tighter dresses that she wore to work. After initial criticisms of her attire met with her resistance, he tried a more balanced approach: "Avery, you're a monster at the gym and I'm proud of you for it. But I wish you'd save some of those sexy outfits for special nights when we go out. It's not that I worry about you, but it drives me crazy to think about other guys staring at you." When he approached Avery in this way, she felt less criticized by Mark and more willing to compromise.

■ *Limit yourself to expressing one main feeling or idea at a time and then give your partner an opportunity to respond.* When one person talks for a long time, the other often stops listening after a while. Limit yourself to just a few sentences and then invite your partner to respond by asking something like "What do you think?" and wait *at least* 10 seconds or more before continuing if your partner remains silent.

■ *Choose your words carefully.* Negative statements that begin with "You always . . . " or "You never . . . " are rarely accurate and usually bring about a defensive response.

■ *Choose your timing.* If you're going to raise a difficult issue or express a painful feeling, try to do it when you're both available and have the emotional energy to have a thoughtful discussion.

■ *Address important feelings as soon as possible.* Don't hold back on expressing difficult feelings so long that they build up inside until you finally explode. To your partner, it will seem as if you've merely over-reacted to a minor incident.

■ *Accept responsibility for your own behaviors that may have contrib-uted to the problem.* Even if you believe your partner is responsible for 90% of a particular problem, search for the 10% of responsibility that is yours. The more you can demonstrate a willingness to accept ownership for your contributions to a problem, the easier it is for your partner to do so as well. For example, although you're never responsible for your partner's bad choices, some of your behaviors might have influenced their decision and it can be helpful to acknowledge them and work to change them.

How Can I Understand My Partner?

Effective communication requires equal parts of expressing your own feel-ings and listening and responding constructively to your partner. Being a good listener can be much harder than being a good speaker, especially when you see things differently. How can you listen to and understand your partner, and how can you best *communicate* that understanding? You need to (1) communicate your willingness to listen up front, (2) respond appropriately while your partner is still speaking, and (3) respond con-structively after your partner has finished.

COMMUNICATING YOUR WILLINGNESS TO LISTEN

People who feel unheard are likely to respond either by disengaging from the conversation or by repeating the message in a louder voice or using more intense language. You can help to avoid these problems by demon-strating your willingness to listen by adopting one of two strategies:

1. Making yourself available when your partner asks to be heard
2. Inviting your partner to talk with you when your partner seems distressed

Making yourself available means eliminating other distractions and offering your full attention. It can be as simple as turning to face your partner and waiting to hear what your partner has to say, or it can be more explicit—turning off the television, silencing and putting away phones, and asking, "What would you like to discuss?" Being available to listen is also communicated by how you present yourself nonverbally. Turn to your partner, relax your facial muscles, adopt a softened or more relaxed physical posture, and lower the volume of your voice when you respond.

Inviting your partner to talk with you when your partner appears distressed requires that you recognize that distress in the first place. Your partner may appear quieter than usual, less spontaneous or responsive to your touch, more irritable, or just more distracted. You can communicate your interest in listening by (1) checking out your partner's feelings, (2) offering to listen to these feelings, and (3) suggesting a time for talking further if necessary.

> When Mariah noticed one evening that Antonio seemed particularly quiet, she tried to pull him out of it by talking about her own day and asking about his, but he offered little in return. Finally she said, "You seem pretty quiet tonight, Antonio, and I can't figure out what's going on. Are you upset about something?" Antonio then told Mariah that he had run into Luke at a meeting and had found it almost unbearable as he recalled Mariah's affair with Luke that had ended six months earlier. Mariah recognized that further discussion was important, but the timing was all wrong because the children were still up and demanding their attention. She responded to Antonio's distress by saying, "I'm sorry. I know you're still upset. Could we talk about this some more after getting the children to bed?"

RESPONDING WHILE YOUR PARTNER IS STILL SPEAKING

While your partner is speaking, it's important to show you're still interested in listening by following these guidelines:

■ *Don't interrupt.* It's hard to listen when your partner is talking about difficult issues, saying things that hurt you or that you disagree with. But one of you has to be willing to listen and demonstrate your understanding first, and we're encouraging you to be the one to do that.

■ *Don't focus on your own response while your partner is speaking.* Your partner isn't going to feel heard if it's clear that you're anxiously awaiting your turn to speak, and if you *are* dying for your chance to talk, it's hard *not* to reveal your impatience through body language.

■ *Avoid challenging, judging, and interpreting.* Avoid asking questions except to seek clarification. For example, it's okay to say, "I'm not sure I understand what you're saying. Could you tell me more about what you mean?" But it won't be helpful to say, "How could you feel that way? Tell me *why* you think that." In fact, as a general rule, "why" questions elicit more defensive or exaggerated statements as your partner feels obligated to justify their position. Similarly, avoid judging or interpreting your partner's thoughts and feelings while listening, for example, avoid responses such as "You've always been insecure—it's not my fault."

■ *Be sure you understand your partner's goal for this discussion.* Does your partner just want to be heard and understood, or does your partner want to solve a problem or reach a decision with you? If you're unsure, ask your partner to clarify.

RESPONDING AFTER YOUR PARTNER HAS FINISHED SPEAKING

The best way to demonstrate that you've heard your partner is to repeat back the thoughts or feelings that your partner has expressed. Various terms describe this process: *mirroring, paraphrasing, reflecting,* and *active listening* are just a few. At the simplest level, you can demonstrate that you've accurately heard your partner by repeating what your partner has said using your partner's original words: "I hear you saying you don't think we have sex often enough and you'd like us to change that." A slightly higher level of responding involves paraphrasing your partner's thoughts or feelings in your own words. For example, "You'd like to make love more often, and you'd like us to explore ways of doing this together. Is that right?" Restating it in your own words might be more difficult or feel slightly riskier, but it also can communicate that you're really trying to understand. See the box below for situations in which active listening can be helpful.

Sometimes your partner's feelings are only implied through tone of voice or body language. When this happens, you might demonstrate your understanding by labeling the implied feeling: "It sounds as though you're feeling frustrated that we're not making love as often as you'd like, and maybe you're feeling hurt that I don't appear as interested in you sexually as before. Is that right?" By checking out your reflection at the end with "Is that right?" you're inviting your partner to confirm or correct your understanding and also avoiding the appearance of mind reading or interpreting.

Reflecting isn't the same as agreeing—it's a way of letting your partner know that you listened and that you understand. And, in fact, one of the most important times to reflect is when you're about to disagree. For example, you might say, "I know you're unhappy with our sex life right now, and you think I'm no longer sexually attracted to you. But actually I'm very attracted to you. I just pull back from you because I still feel too vulnerable when we're close in that way. I don't know how to get rid of those feelings."

Active listening through reflection and validation can be especially helpful when:

- Your partner isn't feeling understood by you.
- You want to demonstrate that you've heard and understood before offering your own thoughts or feelings.
- You're unsure of what your partner is trying to communicate and you want to express your best understanding before asking for clarification.
- You want to focus on your partner's experience and invite them to continue sharing thoughts and feelings.
- Your discussion is getting too heated or escalating into an exchange of complaints and countercomplaints.

Reaching Decisions Together

Chloe and Ava kept going over and over their budget but could never agree on how to get their finances under control. Each discussion ended in a stalemate; Chloe had her preferred solution, and Ava had hers. Each seemed so intent on winning the argument that neither noticed they were losing the broader goal of finding a workable compromise to reduce their frequent quarreling over money. Lingering bitterness from the affair seemed to seep into many of their discussions.

How Do We Reach Decisions Together?

Even when you're doing well at listening and responding to each other's feelings, it's sometimes difficult to reach decisions together. You and your partner may easily get sidetracked. For example, if you're trying to decide whether to replace the washer, as you talked about last month, you might start to discuss how much extra money has already been spent because of the affair. You may get deadlocked on an issue and find it difficult to compromise. Or one of you starts a discussion about a recurrent problem in your relationship, but the other keeps retreating or avoiding the issue.

When you or your partner is upset and you're having trouble communicating, adding more structure to the conversation and using the following guidelines for reaching decisions can be especially helpful.

STATE THE ISSUE WITHOUT BLAME

Often couples get off track because they're unclear about or have forgotten the specific issue they're trying to resolve. At the beginning of your discussion, summarize the issue clearly without anger or blame. For example, try "I'd like us to decide how we're going to handle physical affection and touching each other for now" instead of "We need to talk about how you always want to have sex." If you find yourselves getting off track, try to refocus your discussion by stating "I'm concerned we're starting to get off track. Can we refocus on the specific issue we're trying to resolve?"

CLARIFY WHY THE ISSUE IS IMPORTANT

Partners don't always recognize or understand why an issue is important to the other person, so they don't have a good idea of what a good decision would be. In considering why a particular issue is important to you or your partner, ask yourself these questions: Why is this issue so important? What needs to be taken into account for either of us to be content, and what might either of us be willing to let go?

> Sydney couldn't understand why Brady insisted that he didn't want his parents to know about Sydney's affair. Sydney thought Brady was ashamed of her, and Brady thought Sydney was insisting on telling his parents just to relieve her own conscience. Their discussion moved forward after Brady clarified why this was important to him: "What's most important to me is that you and I try to get our own relationship squared away first. I'm afraid if we tell my parents before we know where we're headed, they'll never get over it, even if we stay together." This helped Sydney explain her own feelings: "I'm not trying to make a confession to your parents just to help myself feel less guilty. But I want to reestablish my honesty with them at some point so that they can still have at least some level of respect for me, despite what I've done. The exact timing isn't that important to me, but being honest with them is." Based on this fuller understanding of what was important to both of them, they then discussed possible solutions and decided to hold off talking to his parents for now, with a commitment to update them at a later time.

FOCUS ON POSSIBLE SOLUTIONS

Couples often spend more time focusing on what's been wrong and who's to blame than on how to change things. You can interrupt the blaming cycle by focusing on what *you* are willing to change, instead of focusing on what you want your partner to change. For example: "I think we're focusing more right now on who's at fault instead of what each of us could do to make this better in the future. How about if I suggest what I think *I* could do to help with this, and then maybe you could give your ideas about what *you* could do?"

Couples often get deadlocked when partners each focus on only one or two of their own preferred solutions. If you find yourselves getting locked into considering only a few possible solutions, try to generate as many possible strategies as you can, even if some ideas seem silly or incomplete. We sometimes encourage structuring this brainstorming process by having one partner write down the different solutions each generates so that they're not forgotten in the heat of the moment and can be reconsidered later in the discussion. Suspending "critical evaluation" of potential solutions as they're first proposed allows new solutions or blends of different solutions to emerge.

DECIDE ON A SOLUTION THAT IS AGREEABLE TO BOTH OF YOU

It's unlikely one solution is going to please both you and your partner equally well. Look for ways to incorporate aspects of proposed solutions from each of you or consider what you both said when discussing why this issue feels important. Work toward an initial solution that both of you are willing to try, even if you're not sure whether it will work in the long run. Take a risk! Then write down specifically what you've agreed on so there are no questions later.

DECIDE ON A TRIAL PERIOD

When you write down the solution, agree on a date for it to begin and on how long you'll try it initially. For certain issues, the decision reached may be "permanent" and won't require a trial period—for example, the decision to end an ongoing affair as a basis for trying to salvage your primary relationship. But agreeing to a trial period for issues that happen repetitively often reduces the discomfort of not knowing in advance whether you could live with that decision in the long run.

> Joel and Mya had always struggled with coordinating their work schedules, but following Joel's affair, she felt determined to do this better as one way to reduce daily stress. Mya had always been responsible for getting their children to school, but on some days this got her to work late and she missed critical meetings. But when Joel offered to take over getting the children dressed and fed in the morning and then driving

them to school, Mya was anxious that he might not be able to handle this, given new additional responsibilities of his own at work. They got unstuck when Joel proposed a 30-day trial period for his taking care of the children in the mornings. If that didn't work, they'd come back and brainstorm some additional strategies.

So, to sum up: Limit discussions of the past to avoid blame; clarify why an issue is important and consider a variety of solutions; compromise, and then compromise some more; and remember that your decisions can always be renegotiated if they're not successful initially.

Preventing Further Damage: What Should We Do When It Gets Too Heated?

Take a Time-Out

Despite your best intentions, there may be times when either you or your partner becomes too emotionally upset to engage in discussions about the affair or other relationship issues constructively. Although such experiences are fairly common among couples struggling to recover from an affair, left unchecked, such escalations can create new and even deeper wounds. For many couples, learning when and how to take a time-out from destructive interactions is the cornerstone of not making things worse.

What is a *time-out*? Essentially, it's an agreement between you and your partner to take a break from interacting when either one of you feels too angry or too fearful to continue constructively. It's like a time-out in a sports game to regain your focus and then resume in a more planful way. Time-outs aren't intended as a way to avoid dealing with difficult issues or as a way to punish your partner for raising them; instead, they offer a strategy for suspending interactions that seem likely to spiral out of control or cause further damage or providing a break when one of you needs time and space to think further on your own.

Using time-outs constructively can sometimes be difficult. The following guidelines should help. Completing Exercise 3.1 will also help you and your partner use time-outs when discussions get too heated.

MONITOR YOUR OWN FEELINGS

You and your partner each need to pay attention to your own feelings and recognize when they're getting so intense that you can't interact productively. Common signs might include yelling or getting louder as you speak, not being able to listen to your partner, experiencing excessive muscle tension or lightheadedness, or even feeling an urge to strike out at your partner.

ACKNOWLEDGE FEELINGS WITHOUT BLAME

When you feel the need to call a time-out, the goal should be to separate so that you can discuss things together more effectively later. Time-outs work best when you can recognize your own escalating anger and call for a time-out by saying something like "I'm getting too upset to talk more now. I think it might be best if we take a 30-minute time-out before continuing."

SHARE THE RESPONSIBILITY

Time-outs also work best when couples agree beforehand that *either* partner can call a time-out, including the partner who may be feeling anxious because of the other one's anger. If your partner's emotions feel frightening or destructive to you but your partner doesn't call for a time-out, acknowledge your own discomfort and request a time-out: "I'm concerned that our discussion is getting too heated and won't be helpful. Let's both take a 30-minute time-out and then try again."

DEVELOP A SHARED PLAN

Time-outs also work better if you develop a plan for how you'll handle them in advance. Once you decide to take a time-out, it usually helps if you and your partner go to separate areas. Before you go to separate areas, agree on (1) how long the time-out will last and (2) when and where you'll get back together. This gives both of you a sense of what to expect and helps to avoid miscommunications such as "I left because I thought you didn't want to see me again tonight."

USE THE TIME-OUT CONSTRUCTIVELY

It's also important to consider what to do and what not to do during a time-out. For example, going over and over the earlier argument in your mind is only likely to maintain or increase your anger or other feelings of distress. Instead, read a book, work on an unfinished task, or calm yourself through meditation or moderate physical exercise. If going for a walk helps to calm you, be sure you let your partner know where you're going and when you'll be back.

Don't do anything during the time-out that could potentially be hurtful to you or to others—for example, drinking alcohol or driving when you're upset. Instead, use the time-out to consider how to interact effectively when you get back together, either thinking about possible solutions to issues you're discussing or trying to clarify your feelings in a nonblaming manner.

COMMON HAZARDS

Although there are many ways that time-outs can go wrong, several patterns are particularly common. First, one partner doesn't honor the other person's request to take a time-out. If either of you insists on "getting the last word," the end is never reached and the escalation continues. Other times one partner fears that the person leaving won't return and tries to block or restrain the person from leaving. That leads to a physical confrontation that can spiral into aggression. This is why it's so important that a time-out called by either partner be implemented immediately.

After the time-out is over, get back together and try discussing the issue again. If you're still not able to discuss the problem without either one of you getting too heated, take another time-out or suggest an alternative time (for example, the next day) to continue your discussion. Don't try to continue if either one of you is feeling emotionally or physically worn out. Be patient, trust the process, and use time-outs to keep things from getting worse so you can come back and try again at a better time.

Write a Letter to Express Your Feelings

In our work with couples struggling to recover from an affair, we often suggest writing a letter as a way of helping partners express their feelings more effectively. Writing a letter allows you to step back from your feelings to gain a broader perspective and to examine your feelings at a deeper level when you're not immediately confronted with your partner's reactions or challenges. Letter writing provides an opportunity to express a more complete picture of what you're experiencing *before* you and your partner get caught up in processing any one particular part of that picture. It provides more opportunity to consider which feelings to emphasize and which ones to omit to get your message across. It's not intended as a strategy to avoid talking to your partner; those conversations will come when the time is better.

Letter writing also increases your opportunity to reflect on your choice of words to express your feelings. How often have you wished you could go back and restate your feelings and express yourself better, only to find that your partner has already latched on to your initial words and that your efforts to "correct" or "amend" your initial message fell on deaf ears? Writing about your feelings in a letter allows you the opportunity to "think before you speak," to consider *how* you want to express yourself, and then to reread what you've written with a "listener's ear" so you can gauge the impact of your message *before* you deliver it. It's important to distinguish between letters written after careful thought and quick notes or emails dashed off as a way of venting feelings. The latter rarely contribute to increased understanding and frequently lead to an escalation of angry exchanges.

Similarly, a letter might be easier for your partner to process because they'll be able to take in a more balanced and complete picture before reacting to any one part of your feelings. A letter allows your partner to deal with their initial reaction to your feelings in private and to gain some perspective before responding. In addition, your partner can choose *when* to read your letter, selecting a time when they're less tired or less distressed.

HOW SHOULD I WRITE THE LETTER?

The guidelines for writing a letter aren't really any different from the guidelines we've already offered for expressing your feelings. Most important is that you try to write a letter that is balanced and focused, and avoids doing further damage. If you're extremely upset or angry, you have two alternatives: (1) wait to write the letter until a later time or (2) write an initial letter that allows you to "vent" your hurt or frustrations at the time, *but destroy the letter afterward*. Letters intended for the purpose of venting that are subsequently "discovered" by your partner can have destructive and long-lasting consequences because they provide a permanent record of your most intense negative feelings. Therefore, we recommend against saving an electronic copy of your letter if you choose to type it rather than write it by hand.

Begin your letter by identifying your feelings and describing how you're finding it difficult to express those feelings constructively face-to-face. Acknowledge that your partner's perspective might be different. Clarify what you're seeking from your partner at this time: Understanding of your feelings? Clarification of your partner's feelings? Reaching a decision together about how to deal with a situation? Keep your letter focused by emphasizing one or two primary feelings and the specific situation giving rise to these feelings. Ask your partner to propose a time and format for responding to your letter—either in a face-to-face discussion or initially in a letter of their own. Exercise 3.2 at the end of this chapter will walk you step by step through the process of writing a constructive, thoughtful letter.

You can also use letter writing at times when you're not able to *listen* or respond to your partner's feelings in the way you'd like. If you and your partner have tried to talk about an issue several times and it just isn't working, consider writing a letter as a way of working through the impasse. Avoid using this letter to express your own thoughts and feelings. Instead, as best you can, validate your partner's views by expressing your understanding of how your partner could come to think or feel that way, given their perspective. Remember: it's not necessary that you agree with your partner—only that you convey your understanding of the thoughts or feelings your partner has expressed.

If subsequent discussions continue to feel hurtful or to spiral out of control as they did initially, exchange letters again, but this time reverse roles so that you can express your feelings and your partner can communicate their understanding of your perspective. Continue to exchange letters, alternating roles as "speaker" and "listener," until each of you feels more understood and more able to respond with understanding to the other. *Above all, remember that letters aren't intended as a substitute for face-to-face discussions.* Rather, they're a first step toward expressing or responding to difficult thoughts and feelings so that your subsequent discussions can be more constructive.

EXERCISES

EXERCISE 3.1 Designing Effective Time-Outs

Write down specific terms for a time-out strategy that you'd like you and your partner to implement if either one of you starts to have feelings that get out of control during your discussion. Your strategy should include the following:

- *Language for calling the time-out.* For example: "I'm starting to feel too angry (or too uncomfortable) to continue this constructively. Let's take a time-out and try again a bit later."

- *Terms of the time-out.* For example: "As soon as either one of us calls a time-out, we'll separate and go to different parts of the house for 30 minutes and then return together to the place where we were having the earlier discussion."

- *Terms for deciding to continue.* For example: "After the time-out we'll check with each other to see whether the other feels ready to continue the discussion. If not, we'll either (1) extend the time-out for an additional 30 minutes or (2) reschedule for a specific day or time later to try again."

Give your proposal for using time-outs to your partner and invite your partner's reactions or suggestions for using time-outs constructively. Revise your proposal as necessary, using both your own and your partner's suggestions. What's most important is agreeing on a plan that will effectively suspend discussions that threaten to spiral out of control and that both you and your partner agree to implement.

EXERCISE 3.2 Writing a Letter to Your Partner

The first part of this exercise involves writing a letter to your partner that describes how the affair has affected your thoughts and feelings about your partner, yourself, and your relationship and how these influence how you're acting right now. In the second part of the exercise, your partner writes a letter in response that conveys an understanding of *your* experience as expressed in your letter. In the last part of the exercise, the two of you discuss your respective letters together.

■ *If you're working through this book with your partner:* This is the ideal process, and you'll exchange *four letters* during this exercise. First, the injured partner will write a letter describing the impact of the affair on their own thoughts, feelings, and behaviors—and then the involved partner will write a letter in response that summarizes their understanding of the injured partner's experience. After an exchange and discussion of these two letters, the involved partner will write a letter describing the impact of the affair on them. Finally, the injured partner will write a letter conveying their understanding of the involved partner's experience.

■ *If you're working through this book alone:* You'll still benefit from writing your own letter detailing the impact of the affair on how you think and feel about your partner, yourself, and your relationship. You may consider sharing this letter with your partner even if you don't expect a response, because your own efforts to describe your experience may promote a better understanding between the two of you. Even if you decide not to share your letter, working through this exercise may help you clarify for yourself the impact of the affair.

In preparing your letter, remember to keep your letter balanced, focused, and constructive. In addition, review the guidelines for expressing feelings summarized on pages 60–62. Choose your words carefully and write about your experience in a way intended to elicit your partner's understanding.

Writing about the Affair's Impact on You

Write a letter to your partner that describes how the affair has affected your thoughts and feelings about your partner, yourself, and your relationship and how they influence your behavior right now. Try to keep your letter somewhat short, perhaps two to five pages.

Describe how the affair has affected your thoughts, feelings, and behaviors regarding your partner. What feelings are you having toward your partner? For example, how distant or close, anxious or secure, angry or loving do you feel? How intense are these thoughts and feelings throughout the day, and how much do they fluctuate moment to moment? How do these thoughts and feelings influence your interactions with your partner? For example, do they cause you to seek closeness, distance, or both at different times?

Describe how the affair has affected your thoughts, feelings, and behaviors regarding yourself. For example, has the affair caused you to struggle with feelings of unattractiveness, depression, or shame? How has the affair influenced how you think about yourself? For example, how confused do you feel about your own actions—both prior to and following the affair? How do your thoughts and feelings influence how you're trying to deal with yourself during this time?

Describe how the affair has affected your thoughts, feelings, and behaviors regarding your relationship. How have your thoughts and feelings about your relationship changed as a consequence of the affair? How have your views of your relationship changed, in either positive or negative ways? Given what's happened, how sure are you about what you wish for your relationship in the long term?

When you've finished writing your letter, put it aside for a day. Then come back and read through it, asking yourself the following questions:

- *Is your letter balanced?* Does it reflect any feelings of hope as well as despair? Any wishes for closeness in addition to impulses to retreat?

- *Is your letter complete?* Have you described the affair's impact on your experience of your partner, yourself, and your relationship?

- *Is your letter constructive?* Does it express your thoughts and feelings in a way that your partner will be able to hear?

If you've answered no to any of these questions, consider waiting another day or two and try revising your letter to communicate more effectively the impact of the affair for you. After you're confident that your letter accurately conveys your experience in each of the three areas we've outlined—and does so in a manner intended to elicit your partner's understanding as constructively as possible—give the letter to your partner and allow them the opportunity to read through it at a separate time and place.

Writing about the Affair's Impact on Your Partner as Your Partner Described It

Write a letter to your partner that reflects how your partner says the affair has affected your partner's thoughts and feelings about you, about them, and about your relationship. This isn't a time to write about your own experience. Rather, it's your opportunity to convey how well you truly understand *your partner's* experience.

Begin your letter by expressing your appreciation for your partner's willingness to share their thoughts and feelings and how they're influencing your partner's interactions with you. Try to summarize the major themes or primary feelings contained in your partner's letter. Specifically, how has the affair affected your partner's thoughts and feelings about you, about them, and about your relationship? Try to use your own words to describe *your partner's* experience as a way of conveying your understanding.

Do the best you can to validate your partner's views by expressing your understanding of how your partner could come to think or feel that way, given their own perspective. Remember: It's not necessary that you agree with your partner—only that you convey your understanding of the thoughts or feelings that they've expressed.

When you've finished writing your letter, put it aside, perhaps for a day or so. Then come back and read through it, asking yourself the following questions:

- *Have you focused on summarizing your partner's experience rather than describing your own?*

- *Have you acknowledged the full range of thoughts and feelings conveyed in your partner's letter?* Have you recognized both positive and negative feelings, if these were expressed? Have you understood and covered how the affair has impacted your partner, their experience of you, and their experience in your relationship?

- *Have you affirmed your partner's perspective?* That is, have you conveyed your own understanding of how your partner could come to think and feel this way, given your partner's particular viewpoint?

After you're confident that your letter conveys your best understanding of your partner's experience, give the letter to your partner and allow them the opportunity to read through it at a separate time and place.

Discussing Your Letters

Once both letters have been exchanged, agree on a time to sit down and discuss them. Begin with the first partner's letter expressing the impact of the affair for them; then proceed to the other partner's letter of understanding. Try to clarify any feelings that are still confusing to either of you. If your discussion begins to feel destructive or gets too heated, take a time-out using the guidelines discussed earlier in this chapter. After you've exchanged and discussed this first set of letters, consider repeating this exercise with the roles reversed. In this second set of letters, the involved partner will write about the affair's impact on them personally, and then the injured partner will write a letter of response that reflects the injured partner's best understanding of the involved partner's experience.

4

How Do We Deal with Others?

Sara couldn't get Kate out of her mind. Rob insisted that their affair was over and that he made sure he and Kate were never alone together at his work site. That wasn't enough for Sara. Rob finally felt pushed to request a move to a different work team. Sara had hoped this arrangement would make her comfortable, but even if she learned to trust Rob again, she would never trust Kate. The only solution in Sara's mind was for Rob to find different employment. Rob initially resisted but finally gave in to Sara's ultimatum and resigned.

A slow economy made it hard for Rob to find another job with equal pay or status, so he took a less prestigious job with a significant pay cut. He resented Sara for "forcing" him to change jobs as a way of "punishing" him for the affair. He felt fully justified in pushing her to return to work to make up for his pay cut, even though he and Sara had initially agreed that Sara would stay home during their daughter's preschool years. Sara's anger toward Rob grew day by day. Not only had he betrayed her as a husband, but now he had forced her to betray their daughter as well. Sara's mother and sister knew about the details of Rob's affair and resented him greatly for it—they always thought she should leave him, so they were hostile to him during family gatherings, creating tension for everyone. Rob's and Sara's bitterness toward each other festered. After two years, they concluded there was little between them to salvage and ended their marriage in a bitter divorce.

How should you deal with your partner's interactions with the outside affair person? Should you and your partner confront the person together?

Should you trust your partner to end it on their own? Should you insist on no further contact, even if that means switching jobs? What if your partner's views on these issues differ from yours?

Did Sara and Rob make a good decision? Could their marriage have been saved if they had come up with another way to limit Rob's contact with Kate to help Sara feel secure? Sara had confided in her mother and sister for emotional support right after the affair happened, but those disclosures created issues down the line for Sara and Rob when they were trying to save their relationship. Was Sara wise to share details of the affair with her family?

Although an affair affects you and your partner most directly, it may also impact your other relationships. Each of you now must decide whom to tell about the affair—and what to tell. How will you respond if others ask you about what's happening? What do you want, if anything, from other people? Although there are no absolute answers to most of these questions, some general principles can guide you in making such decisions.

How Do We Decide Whom to Tell about the Affair?

You may have to tell some people about the affair or, more generally, that your relationship is struggling. For example, your boss might need to know some amount of information about why you can't work with a colleague any longer, or your child's daycare worker may need to understand why your child seems so anxious these days. However, you may not need to disclose the affair per se. What you choose to share can range from nothing to almost everything. At times, you may feel you should tell some people a great deal, such as your closest friend with whom you always share your deepest secrets. And if you need help or support—say, from a sibling whom you count on to be there for you—you'll have to explain why. The important factor in deciding whom to tell is *to be clear and honest with yourself about why you're talking to that person and what you decide to tell them.* You can always share more later, but you can't undo what you've already shared.

This means exploring *all* the motives you might have, not just the "good" ones. You might believe your children deserve to know what's happened because it affects them. But is there a part of you that wants to punish your partner or get your children on your side? Are you pushing your partner to tell the boss "for the welfare of the company," when your secret hope is that the outside person will be fired? Are you planning on sending an anonymous letter to the outside person's partner because it feels like the "right thing," when what you really want is to see their relationship in a shambles just like yours? It's not hard to come up with "good" reasons for telling someone about the affair when there are additional motives that may be less virtuous. But acting on your impulse to get back at your partner or the outside person often has negative consequences in the long term.

Once you know for sure why you want to tell someone about the affair, also think carefully about whether this person is appropriate to turn to for this purpose. For example, should you turn to your children for emotional support while going through this crisis—even if they're now adults? Is it appropriate to ask a couple that you two see together to support you individually or take sides against your partner? Suppose you and your partner eventually decide to remain together. If you turned to a family member for advice on getting through this difficult time, might that person forever resent your partner for hurting you? Should you first contact a mental health professional, a religious or spiritual counselor, or some other person outside of your personal life instead? Someone who can guide you confidentially? *Identifying what you need and finding an appropriate person to meet that need is critical to the recovery process.*

How Do We Deal with the Outside Affair Person?

Whether the affair has ended or not, the outside person is a major part of the trauma you've experienced, and you might view that person as an ongoing threat. The most important issue to address regarding the outside person is how to set boundaries around your relationship and protect it from further intrusion. Without appropriate boundaries, you won't be able to create the sense of safety necessary to move forward as a couple. Continued interactions between your partner and the outside person can feel threatening, may increase the likelihood that the affair will rekindle, and can lead to ongoing emotional turmoil for everyone. But limiting or eliminating contact can be difficult because the outside person may pursue continued contact even though the affair is over, or because the affair hasn't ended yet. This can be even more challenging when the involved partner and the other person work together, are part of the same core friend group, or are part of each other's everyday life in another way. What these boundaries look like for you might vary—for example, is it okay to allow contact in some ways but not others, or does all contact need to end? Maybe you decide against any in-person meetings, but what about responding to text messages, social media posts, or other ways of interacting digitally? These decisions that you need to make together might not be as simple as they seem.

You can address these complications by keeping the following guidelines in mind:

- The clearer and firmer the boundaries, the better for your relationship.

- Don't make agreements you can't keep or will resent.

- Consider in-person contact as well as contact over various media and technology (for example—texts, emails, or social media).

- Discussing these boundaries is a process that takes time, and your decisions may change as time passes.

You and your partner need to have a series of conversations in which you clarify the current status of the relationship with the outside person, express how each of you feels about continued interaction and whether the outside person is willing to let go, and decide on what boundaries to set. *These discussions and negotiations can include some of the most difficult initial issues that couples address when an affair becomes known.* The injured partner will find it painful even to consider possible further contact with the outside person, and the involved partner may have to deal with guilt, shame, anger, or sadness without being permitted to have or express those feelings.

Because these discussions can be so upsetting, some couples avoid them. Some partners believe that if the affair is over they don't need to discuss the outside person. In our experience, however, this kind of avoidance generally doesn't work. *The outside person's continued presence is a critical threat, and you two need to discuss what specific boundaries to set.*

What Boundaries Should We Set If the Affair Has Ended?

> Derek's affair with Rich was supposed to end two months ago, but Rich was so devastated by the idea of losing him that Derek reluctantly agreed that they could be "just friends." But when Derek didn't return his advances when they met, Rich was hurt, enraged, and started calling Derek at home every night. When Derek blocked his calls and tried to cut off contact completely, Rich began sending texts and then leaving notes for Derek's partner, with explicit details of the affair. Everything the couple had done to try to save their relationship fell apart in the constant arguments over how to end Rich's persistent intrusions.

SET CLEAR, STRONG BOUNDARIES FOLLOWING THE AFFAIR

The clearer and stronger the boundaries and the less interaction with the outside person, the better for your relationship. *Trying to remain friends with someone after an affair becomes known rarely works; at least one of the three people in this triangle is likely to find the arrangement unacceptable.* Continued interactions with the outside person will just keep reopening painful thoughts and feelings from the affair and can block any progress toward restoring a sense of security for the injured partner.

Continued interaction doesn't serve the involved partner well either when the goal is to end the affair and move on. Contact with the outside person can rekindle positive feelings and create confusion over important relationship decisions. Moreover, the involved partner may worry about how these meetings will be experienced by either their partner or the outside person. Continuing any kind of relationship can mislead the outside person into believing that the involved partner really doesn't want to end the affair.

Sometimes the involved partner might argue that cutting off all contact is too extreme—that they've agreed to end the affair and that's enough. However, if that's your perspective, consider that affairs often develop through small interactions that build over time, even if specific interactions seem harmless. For example, collaborating on work projects, attending group lunches, or exercising together—even if you're just friends—can lead to feelings. Ending these types of interactions with someone you've felt close to or been involved with helps you avoid the likelihood of things slowly resuming, even when you don't mean for them to.

The bottom line is this: Continued interactions with the outside person usually keep someone or everyone in continued turmoil.

You and your partner will need to establish clear expectations regarding any future contact—how an interaction might come about and how to address it. You'll need to decide whether *any type of communication* is acceptable, as well as whether *any setting for interaction* is acceptable. Exercise 4.1 will help you do this. For example, is a phone conversation okay, but not face-to-face contact? Is texting or emailing acceptable? For most people, the clear answer to all of these questions is "No, nothing is acceptable." However, at times this response is unrealistic, at least right away. For example, if your partner and the outside person work together and the affair has just become known, it might be unrealistic to say "Never speak to that person again about anything." That's why the *setting for interactions* needs to be considered. Even if the involved partner and outside person work together, as a couple you may decide that for now group interaction in a business meeting is acceptable, but one-on-one meetings are not.

Implied in these examples is a third factor: the *topic or focus* of what is discussed during the interactions and what types of interactions are acceptable. Some couples set a boundary that there's to be no discussion of feelings or anything personal with the outside person, but necessary communications about work or about ending the relationship are acceptable for a short time. Any conversations between the involved partner and outside person about how much they miss or care about each other create a high-risk situation. Self-disclosure of feelings leads to more self-disclosure, which then leads to greater feelings of intimacy. Behaviors that may have been acceptable (and seemed harmless) between the injured partner and outside person *before* the affair often are no longer acceptable because they're now high risk for reinvolvement. This may include small physical behaviors such as greeting hugs or "high-fives," communications such as "happy birthday" texts once a year, or even brief interactions on social media. If your partner is behaving in positive ways with the person they've had an affair with, feelings of emotional connection are likely to follow. In other words, previous boundaries may need to be reconsidered and revised—your relationship and interactions with others can't just go back to how they were before.

At times, some kind of interaction with the outside person may be needed to establish the ground rules. As a couple, you should decide on the message and mode of delivery, such as an email message signed by you as a couple. After Diego told Elena about his affair, they decided to write an email message together, which Diego then sent:

"I've told my wife, Elena, about our affair and that I've decided to end it. We're going to work on our relationship. I know this decision may be painful for you, but I've given it a lot of thought, and that is what I'm going to do. I'm asking you not to call or text me or come to see me; just send me a reply saying you've received this message. In a couple of days, I'll contact you to consider whether we can meet in some public setting to say goodbye. After that meeting, I want to ask that we have no further contact of any sort. I need to move on with my life and work on my marriage. Diego."

MAKE REALISTIC AGREEMENTS

Promising to limit interactions with the outside person and then not doing so creates further betrayals and undermines any efforts to restore trust. Therefore, *agree only to what you know you can do*, even if that means taking it a day at a time and then renegotiating as time passes. It's far better for involved partners to be honest throughout this process than to agree to something but then break the agreement behind their partner's back, creating additional betrayals.

Although Antonne wanted Jazmin to end all contact with Sam, Jazmin felt too ambivalent about her relationship with Antonne to end the affair immediately. She knew she couldn't in truth agree to no contact. She summoned up her nerve to express these feelings to Antonne. After some painful negotiation, they agreed she could communicate with Sam via text or email, but she needed to let Antonne know what she was saying. They also agreed that she would maintain this kind of contact only *for a limited time while she was working with an individual therapist on deciding what she wanted to do. At the end of the trial period, they would reassess the situation and Jazmin would have to make a decision.*

VIEW SETTING LIMITS AS AN ONGOING PROCESS

You may not be certain about how you'll react over time to the limits you've set, so you might need to view limit setting as an ongoing process with continuous evaluation and possible renegotiation. This is particularly important if the affair hasn't yet ended. If you discovered your partner's ongoing affair, you may have demanded that they end all forms of interaction with the other person from that moment forward. Your partner might have agreed, only to fail to keep the agreement. Rarely will someone instantly end a meaningful relationship without any further contact with the other person. So discuss between the two of you what's realistic, what the involved partner needs to do to end the affair, and how to structure any future interactions that do occur.

Obviously, the involved partner shouldn't use this recommendation as an excuse to continue an affair or other interactions with the outside person. If you've decided to end an affair, end it as quickly and definitely as possible. Your focus needs to be on your relationship and attending to your partner. *Take responsibility for establishing limits and arrange your life so you can adhere to them.* There may be moments when your warm feelings for the outside person return. But establishing and respecting strong, consistent boundaries can help you get through those times.

When the Affair Has Ended

- Set clear limits on any future contact.
- Be specific about how the involved partner will tell the injured partner when those limits have been violated.
- Agree on a plan for responding if the outside person initiates contact.
- If circumstances such as work require some continued contact, set clear limits on the setting and content of these interactions.

How Do We Respond If the Outside Person Makes Contact?

Even when an affair has ended and your partner faithfully honors the limits set for interacting with the outside person, you need to decide together what to do if there's a chance meeting or one initiated by the outside person. *The most important principle is for the involved partner to inform the injured partner of any such interactions and disclose what happened— however the meeting came about.*

> "The last thing in the world I want to do is tell Claire that Molly texted me," Carter protested. "Claire and I are doing better, so why rock the boat by bringing that up? I didn't respond to Molly's text, so why not let sleeping dogs lie?"

Carter's reaction is understandable, but there are important reasons to tell Claire about the text message. First, failing to disclose it continues deceit and secrecy and works against Carter's pledge to rebuild a truthful relationship with Claire, whether she finds out or not. And if Claire does learn about the contact, their attempts at rebuilding trust are damaged even more deeply. Finally, there's probably nothing Carter can do that will be more powerful to rebuild trust than to share this information. Disclosing interactions that occurred with the outsider can be painful in the short run but usually rebuilds trust in the long run. Therefore: *If you want to rebuild a trusting relationship with your partner, disclose interactions with the outside person, no matter how trivial these interactions may seem or how much turmoil such disclosures may initially create.* Of course, you and your partner want to be realistic in following this principle. If you work with the outside person, you and your partner might agree that you don't discuss every time you receive a group email or sit far apart in a large group meeting with the outside person present. The principle is to disclose any interactions that might be of a personal nature and not to shy away from telling your partner about them. You and your partner can decide what makes sense and change these agreements as time passes.

The flip side of this advice involves the injured partner's response to receiving such information. Learning that your partner and the outside person have had some kind of contact almost always feels threatening and painful. But when the contact was initiated by the outside person and beyond your partner's control, lashing out punishes rather than strengthens your partner's efforts to risk addressing difficult feelings for the sake of rebuilding trust. If the interaction results from behaviors of the outside person, it's still okay to express feelings of anxiety or anger, but also let your partner know that you're not holding them responsible for the *current* exchange. In other words, distinguish between the hurt or anger you have from the affair itself and your feelings about the recent interaction with the outside person that your partner is describing now.

You may also need to take whatever steps are necessary to stop the outside person from unwanted intrusions into your relationship. Partners may decide to act together—for example, by writing and signing a letter from both partners, sending a joint email message, making a joint phone call, or asking to meet together with the person in a public setting. Unfortunately, at times such messages fall on deaf ears. An outside person who refuses to let go may attempt to destroy your relationship, seduce the partner, threaten to kill themselves, or threaten the injured partner or a member of the family. Take such threats seriously and consider getting outside assistance. We've worked with couples who've had to threaten legal action to stop harassment or contact the police to issue a restraining order. In extreme cases, we've known of couples who have switched jobs or moved to another community to get away from someone who simply would not give up on an affair.

When the Outside Person Doesn't Want to Let Go

- Discuss additional ways to emphasize to the outside person that the affair is over.

- Examine possible "mixed messages" to the outside person and make sure they're not sent anymore.

- When these strategies fail, seek assistance in limiting contact—from supervisors at work or through legal action if necessary.

- In extreme circumstances, consider changing jobs or moving to another community.

WHAT IF THE AFFAIR HAPPENED ONLINE OR DIDN'T INVOLVE
JUST ONE PERSON?

We've discussed how infidelity involves important violations of boundaries in areas that typically are reserved just for the couple, often involving a sexual or intimate way of interacting with an outside person. However, it's also possible that your partner may not have cheated on you with one specific person that they know in real life, but instead they've engaged in online activities with one or more other persons in ways that make you uncomfortable or seem like your boundaries have been violated. For example, your partner may watch pornography or view sexual content you find inappropriate or inconsistent with your values. Or they may repeatedly fantasize about others during your sexual exchanges (which you've discovered when they accidentally spoke someone else's name during sex), or they've engaged with sex workers in video chat rooms or on the phone. For many couples, these activities aren't acceptable and are considered cheating. For some couples, however, they're not necessarily boundary violations and may even be acceptable. What's important is that every couple must decide for themselves what boundaries are important to maintain—regardless of context (in person versus digital), level of engagement (viewing versus actively participating), and whether the violation involves a single individual or more than one. If those boundaries are crossed, the couple then needs to decide what's necessary to reestablish security and trust in those domains.

What Boundaries Should We Set If the Affair Is Still Going On?

If you've found out about your partner's ongoing affair, and your partner doesn't realize you know, confronting your partner about the affair and deciding what to do is the first critical step. In our experience, ignoring a partner's affair in the hope that it will end on its own is unlikely to work. If you've already confronted your partner and they've refused to end the affair at the present time, most likely it's because they're uncertain whether to continue your relationship or the relationship with the outside person. Sometimes a person doesn't actually want to leave their primary relationship for the other person, but the affair with the outsider is so gratifying in some ways that the person doesn't want to end it until absolutely necessary. If this is the case in your relationship, we recommend that you do the following: *Make it necessary.* As the injured partner, clearly state your unwillingness to accept an ongoing affair in the long run and be adamant that your partner work toward difficult decisions about how to resolve this. Work toward firm limits, but don't give premature ultimatums or ones that can't be honored.

What should you do if your partner seems unwilling to end an affair? No single answer to this question works equally well for everyone, and we urge you to ignore anyone who offers a definitive answer. The primary risk of allowing a partner to continue an affair is that some involved partners will settle into long-term or semipermanent indecision. We've worked with couples who had been in this state of indecision for five years or longer before seeking counseling. Unless absolutely necessary, some involved partners simply don't decide between their primary relationship and the outside person.

The major risk in pushing for a decision is that the involved partner may decide to end your relationship when you still want to salvage it. If your relationship with your partner feels particularly bad, and your partner's affair seems particularly important or rewarding, your partner may indeed end your relationship before you have an opportunity to rebuild it, even declaring that your forcing the issue caused this outcome.

Alternatively, for some injured partners forcing the issue is a way of regaining a sense of control when life has felt very much out of control. Many people find it emotionally abusive when a partner continues an affair, and forcing a decision is a way of ending the mistreatment. If the couple's relationship survives after forcing this decision, then the injured partner has clearly established that such violations of boundaries will not be tolerated in the future.

However, if it appears, for whatever reasons, that a partner's affair is going to continue for some time, it's still important to discuss what types of boundaries to set regarding the outside person. Some couples separate while an affair is ongoing, and if you do, it's important to make short-term agreements while you decide together about the future of your relationship. For example, you may need to decide how to handle your finances,

When the Affair Is Still Going On

- Distinguish between intermediate- and long-term goals. Be realistic about what to expect in the short term.

- Agree on a time frame for the involved partner to reach a decision regarding the affair.

- Define the limits, if any, on the nature of continued contact with the outside person.

- Develop specific guidelines for communicating with each other about either partner's contact with the outside person.

- Be clear about next steps to pursue once the involved partner decides to end the affair or if either of you decides to end your relationship.

how to interact either separately or together around your children's activities, and what boundaries apply with the outside person while you and your partner are separated.

If your partner refuses to end an affair but is also asking not to end your relationship, you face a painful dilemma. You and your partner have to live with the consequences of your decisions, so be very careful as you consider any well-intended advice from others. It can be just as reasonable to decide to stay for now as to push for a decision. *Take the time you need; making a major life decision when you're upset, tired, or worn down can be risky.* At these times many people find that a professional trained to help with difficult life decisions gives them a useful outside perspective.

What Do We Tell the Children and How Do We Interact with Them?

Maggie was devastated by Liam's affair, and she was determined that he wouldn't get away with it. She told both of their teenage daughters what their father had done and waited to see their outrage. She wasn't prepared for the depth of their hurt and confusion. Years later, Maggie's older daughter confessed that knowing about her father's affair still haunted her in her own romantic relationships, *and she described how much she had hated being caught between him and her mother.*

If you have children and one of you has been involved in an affair, you've probably been asking yourself, "What do we tell the children?" Children of most ages are aware when there's heightened tension between their parents. You and your partner may argue more often or intensely, or either one of you may show various signs of your distress. It seems important to say or do something, but what?

In deciding what to say and do, make your children's well-being your top concern. Beyond that, make the guidelines in the box below your mantra; refer to them often as a reminder after reading the explanations that follow. Exercise 4.2 will also help you reach decisions about how to interact with your children about the affair.

Help Your Children Maintain Loving Relationships with Both Parents

When the relationship between you and your partner is disrupted, your children need the security of strong relationships with both parents. You may want a chance to explain your side of the story, or you may feel your partner doesn't deserve your children's love and affection. When such thoughts cross your mind, always come back to principle number one: *If it's not in your children's best interest, it's not the right choice.* Research indicates that children can endure conflicts between their parents, including

Guidelines for Dealing with Children

- Help your children maintain caring and loving relationships with both parents.
- Say only what is necessary.
- Adjust what you say according to your children's ages and levels of development.
- Minimize the disruption to your children's lives.
- Avoid having your children take care of you during this crisis.

divorce, if they can maintain loving relationships with both parents and not have to choose sides between them.

Say Only What Is Necessary

A key question for many parents is whether to tell the children explicitly that one partner has had or is having an affair. We don't advocate that you lie to your children, but consider carefully what to share and what to keep to yourself. If many people know about the affair, including your children's friends or their parents, and your children are likely to learn about it, you may want to tell them yourselves so that you have some control over what they hear and how they hear it.

It's important to talk with children, however, when there's significant distress in your relationship. They're likely to experience that *something* is wrong but may be confused without additional information. Consequently, it's important to acknowledge that the two of you aren't getting along and are unhappy with each other right now. It also can be helpful for children to know what will change and what will remain the same. For example, you may want to let them know that you might not be doing as many things together as a family but will continue to live together.

In many instances there's no clear reason why the children need to know about an affair unless it's likely to become public knowledge. Just as you'd be unlikely to tell your children about difficulties in your sexual relationship, you don't necessarily need to tell them about the *specific basis* of other relationship problems. What your children need help in understanding is the general magnitude of their parents' conflicts and what's likely to change or remain the same in their own lives. *Remember that the **most** important information your children need is that both parents still love them very much.*

Adjust What You Say to Your Children's Ages and Levels of Development

Whatever you say to your children, use language that they can understand based on their age and level of development. For example, if you're speaking to a 10-year-old and have decided it's essential to share about an outside person, you might say, "Your dad isn't sure he wants to continue being married to me. He's found someone else that he cares about a lot, so let me tell you what's going to happen." If your children are far apart in age, you may want to talk with each child separately so that you can adjust what you say according to each child's level of development.

Not only must you decide *what* to tell your children, but you also have to decide *how* to tell them. Usually if you're telling your children about your relationship difficulties, it's beneficial if you and your partner talk with them together. That can prevent either one of you from presenting the situation in a blaming way and can avoid the inevitable differences in your accounts that could lead to confusion for your children or their feeling caught in the middle between you.

Some couples decide to have each parent talk with the children separately—either because they're so angry with each other that they risk having an argument in front of the children or because one partner fears becoming too distressed to get through a discussion if the other partner is present. If you decide to talk to your children separately, make sure you've discussed what each of you will say, how you'll handle certain issues that might come up, and how you'll try to avoid blaming each other or putting your children in the middle of your own struggles.

Minimize the Disruption to Your Children's Lives

When you talk to your children about your relationship problems, they may become worried or sad. Some experience their distress through anger, or it results in poor school performance, whereas others seem almost indifferent to the family crisis. Regardless of how your children respond, recognize that the upcoming months may be very difficult for them. As you've experienced yourself, loss of control and unpredictability are usually frightening. *Do whatever you can to maintain your children's typical daily routines.* At the same time, be sure to talk with your children about any significant changes, particularly any changes in living arrangements, as well as both parents' ongoing participation in meals, school activities, community activities, or family vacations.

Avoid Having Children Take Care of You during This Crisis

During this difficult time, you may need lots of support, both emotional and practical. Although it's certainly appropriate for your children to show care and concern for you, they shouldn't be the ones you turn to for support or advice about your relationship, even if they're grown. *Turning to your children for emotional support often forces them to choose between their two parents, an unfair choice for you to impose at any age.*

Aside from emotional support, when people are under a lot of stress, they often need extra practical support or help with various tasks. Although it might be appropriate to ask children to help out more during these difficult times, be careful not to overdo it. Having children who help out can be wonderful, but make certain that the children continue to be children, functioning in a way that's appropriate for their age and level of individual development. You also might want to consider whether your children might benefit from a professional counselor during this time to give them a safe place to explore their own reactions to the situation.

What Do We Tell Family Members and Friends?

In a fit of rage, Luis told his family about Daniela's affair. As he had hoped, his family rallied around him in support and in anger at her betrayal. However, in the following weeks, Luis decided that he really loved Daniela and didn't want to leave her. As they both worked to rebuild their relationship, his family's support turned to anger at Luis. They couldn't understand how he could take her back and told him he was weak and foolish. Daniela was furious at their treatment of both her and Luis, and they both ended up feeling isolated from his family.

You might tell family members or friends about an affair because you think they should know or you want their support. Consider carefully who, if anyone, should know about your current difficulties and exactly what they should know. You may decide to tell family members and friends that you're having difficulties, but not share with them that one of you has had an affair. This might be particularly complicated if other family members are living with you and have picked up on the tension and distress between you and your partner. Consider whether you need to share any information with them about what's going on—and how much to share—so they don't say something unintentionally in front of the children that could make things worse. In other cases, you may have a trusting relationship with a family member or friend whose assistance or advice regarding the affair could be quite valuable. The guidelines summarized in the box at the bottom of this page are discussed more thoroughly on the next few pages. Exercise 4.3 will also help you reach decisions about talking with others about the affair.

Will Telling This Person Damage a Long-Term Relationship with My Partner?

Particularly if you're the injured partner, you may want to tell your parents, siblings, or friends about what your partner has done and the hurtful effects on you. Sharing such information is one way of gaining support. But before talking with family or friends about your partner's affair, think about how your comments might impact their relationship with your partner in the future. If you and your partner restore your relationship and stay together, will your family member or friend also be able to rebuild a relationship with your partner? Despite their best intentions, family members are sometimes unable to move beyond anger or resentment toward a partner who brought such pain to someone they love. And if you have other struggles with your partner in the future, it may be difficult to discuss them with your family or friends because they no longer support your relationship. Moreover, sometimes the involved partner has such deep embarrassment or shame that it's difficult to interact with the other person's family or friends in the future.

If you've already talked with a family member or friend about the affair

---

Guidelines for Talking with Others

- Will telling this person about the affair damage their relationship with my partner?

- Will this person respect my request for confidentiality?

- What specifically do I want from this person?

- If I'm looking for advice, can this person take a balanced perspective?

and your partner knows you've done so, it can sometimes be helpful if you and your partner get together with that person and attempt to rebuild the friend's or family member's relationship with your partner. Even if you and your partner decide to separate or divorce, it may be important for your partner to maintain a cordial relationship with your family, particularly if you have children. So think carefully about the long-term implications of talking with family or close friends about the affair, recognizing that your own feelings about your partner and your relationship may change in unexpected ways over the coming months.

Will This Person Respect My Request for Confidentiality?

It's important that you also consider whether your family member or friend will honor your wish for confidentiality. In many families or friendship circles, there's an informal rule that important personal information can and should be shared. Often this information is conveyed in this way: "Mary told me something very confidential, and she doesn't want anyone else to know. But I thought you needed to know. So don't say anything about it to anyone, okay?" If people are likely to find out, then you may wish to tell them directly rather than having the information presented secondhand, with all the possibilities of misinformation and distortion. Concerns about confidentiality are one reason that many people decide to talk about the details of what they're experiencing to professionals instead.

What Specifically Do I Want from This Person?

Are you looking for emotional support, for advice, or for other assistance with practical issues or demands? For example, with friends or family members, what you may need is a good shoulder to lean on, someone who understands you and will just listen. There are probably other people whom you're likely to seek out for advice or strategic assistance. For example, you might want the name of a mental health professional or some other counselor with whom to talk about your current difficulties, or you may want professional advice from a financial consultant or attorney. You might approach a family member or friend for assistance with specific tasks that aren't being accomplished during this time of relationship crisis, such as help with child care, meals, or transportation. Be clear about what you're looking for—with yourself and with the person you're talking to about your situation—and share only what is needed.

Can This Person Take a Balanced Perspective and Not Just Take My Side?

Family members and friends typically see it as their responsibility to support you during a crisis and to see things from your perspective. It's unlikely they can be totally objective in how they view or respond to your situation, but it's important that their perspective is balanced. We've seen many examples in which family and friends basically tell an injured partner, "Ditch the jerk and make life as miserable as possible for them." It's easy to focus on the pain resulting from this affair right now, but you may lose sight of what your relationship has provided in the past and what it might be able to provide at some point again in the future. Only you—not your family member or friend—will have to live with the consequences of whatever long-term decisions you make about your relationship. *So be very careful about placing too much weight on any advice you receive, no matter how well intended.*

Also be aware that if you seek advice from family or friends, they may be upset with you if you don't follow it. Ask them to respect your final decision, even if it's not consistent with their advice. Your family and friends can support you in many valuable ways through this difficult time. If you're thoughtful about the friends and family members to whom you turn, if you think about what you want from each of these relationships and carefully consider both the short- and long-term consequences of disclosing the affair, you can benefit from being supported by people who care about you.

Look over the exercises on the following pages and consider which of these may apply to you. Some of the challenges you're facing depend on the unique circumstances of your own situation, such as whether the affair has ended and whether you have children. If you and your partner are working through this book together, each of you should think about your own views and then share your thoughts and feelings about these issues and decide what to do. If you're working through the book alone and your partner is unwilling to discuss these issues, you'll need to decide on your own what to do, but whenever possible, inform your partner about your plans.

EXERCISES

EXERCISE 4.1 How Do We Deal with the Outside Person?

In setting limits with the outside person, consider three different issues: (1) the method of communicating with the outside person, (2) the settings for interactions, and (3) what is to be discussed. You might also need to take action to prevent this person from interfering in your lives.

Method of Communication

Discuss various ways of communicating between the outside person and the individual who had the affair and decide what is acceptable. For example:

> "We've agreed that you're not to have any form of contact with the other person whatsoever. If the outside person contacts you by email or texts, you'll ignore it. If that person calls, you'll hang up immediately. If they persist, you'll block them from being able to reach you. If you run into each other, you won't acknowledge them or speak."

If the affair is ongoing, you still need to discuss what limits are acceptable for now and how these limits will change over time. For example:

> "We've agreed you'll have two months to decide whether you plan to end that relationship or ours. In the meantime, you're not to take any phone calls here or send email or text messages from home. You've also agreed to be honest and inform me about your contacts with the outside person. In one week, we'll reconsider whether I can live with this arrangement."

Settings for Communication

Given the circumstances, some interaction with the outside person may be unavoidable. Discuss whether it's acceptable for your partner to interact with the outside person in certain settings and what limits to set. For example:

"Because you work with this person, I know you can't totally avoid them. We've agreed that it's okay to be in a group meeting with that person, but that you won't have any meetings with just the two of you, either in the office or outside."

Content of Communication

If you and your partner agree that some forms of communication with the outside person are acceptable or necessary, you need to specify what will and will not be discussed with the outside person. Conversations about business are quite different from those about how much you care about each other. For example:

"We've agreed that you can discuss business issues, but that's all. You're not to discuss your former relationship with each other, how you feel about each other, or how you're doing emotionally."

Additional Steps to Set Limits

You may find that the outside person is reluctant or unwilling to stay out of your lives. If so, you might need to take additional action such as consulting with a lawyer, changing jobs, or even moving to another community. For example:

"We'll contact our lawyer and ask her to send a letter to the outside person, informing them that they're to have no further contact with any member of our family. If the person doesn't comply, our next step will be to contact the police regarding harassment."

EXERCISE 4.2   What Do We Tell Our Children and How Do We Minimize the Impact on Them?

What and How to Tell the Children

Decide what you need to convey to your children and how you want to communicate it. For example:

"We've agreed to meet with the children together and to let them know that we're having some difficulties in getting along right now, but that we're getting some help in trying to make things better.

We've also agreed not to make any direct or indirect comments about the affair itself."

Minimizing Disruptions to the Family Routine

Discuss how the current distress in your relationship could affect family routines or other aspects of your children's lives and reach decisions about how to minimize these disruptions. For example:

"We've agreed to have family meals together and for both of us to participate in our children's school and extracurricular activities. We've agreed during these times not to discuss the affair and to interact as constructively as possible. For now, we've agreed to wait one month before reaching a decision about how to deal with summer vacation."

EXERCISE 4.3 Whom Else Do We Tell?

Decide whom you want to talk with about the affair and how much detail you want to disclose. Be clear about what you want from the individual, whether confiding in this person could hinder your recovery as a couple in the long term, and whether the person is likely to respect your wishes for confidentiality. For example:

"I want to talk with my best friend about the affair because I value her judgment and her emotional support, and I trust her not to tell anyone else. If other friends ask me about what's going on, I will only say that we're having some relationship problems but are working on them. For now, I would prefer that neither my family nor yours know about our relationship problems. I'm willing to reevaluate this decision a month from now."

5

How Do We Care for Ourselves?

*Emma's life turned upside down after she discovered that her part-
ner, Sierra, had secretly renewed her involvement with a prior girl-
friend. She couldn't sleep, and her emotions swung wildly from
numbness to anger or despair. Normally Emma turned to Sierra for
help, but now Sierra seemed like a stranger. Emma had no idea how
to get her emotions and life back under control.*

*Sierra also lay awake at night, tormented by thoughts of the
pain she had caused Emma. But she was also furious at Emma for
having neglected her so completely this past year. When they tried
to discuss what had happened, the pain and anger each felt seemed
so unbearable that they would often end up losing control and
screaming at each other. This only made things worse, but neither
of them knew how to break the cycle.*

The days and weeks following the discovery of an affair are often chaotic and emotionally traumatic. You can barely get through the day and
manage the work you have to do. You need all the strength you can get—
but taking care of yourself seems even more difficult and perhaps a lower
priority. But know this:

🖋 Healthy self-care is critical to recovery—not just for
yourself, but for your relationship.

First, adequate self-care is essential to combat the effects of stress. The
discovery or disclosure of an affair typically creates high, sustained stress

for both partners. Just when you most need additional emotional, physical, and social strength, you may be least likely to engage in behaviors designed to renew these resources. For example, you may be exhausted and need a good night's sleep, but instead you find yourself lying awake at night, worrying about the future or reviewing every detail of the past to try to understand what went wrong. Lack of sleep brings more exhaustion and less resilience. Or your worry about other people discovering the problems you and your partner are having may lead you to avoid friends and family. If so, being more isolated socially may only increase your emotional distress. You can end up feeling particularly isolated if you've previously counted on your partner for emotional support. So for now you may find yourself needing to take care of yourself in ways you haven't needed to do before.

Second, failure to take care of yourself will inevitably make things worse. Research on the mind–body connection clearly shows that lack of sleep, poor nutrition, and inadequate social support all lead to increased emotional and physical reactions that can be unhealthy, which in turn increases the likelihood that you will not handle difficult discussions well. *If you don't take care of yourself during this recovery process, you're likely to find both you and your relationship getting worse.* Healthy self-care helps to build up your resilience and strengthen you for the hard work that lies ahead in rebuilding your life after the affair.

How Do I Get Through the Day?

Attending to Emotional Needs

Anxiety, depression, and anger take a toll on your physical health, get in the way of meeting your day-to-day responsibilities, and often intrude on your interactions with your partner in ways that make recovery more difficult. Strategies for making times of emotional upset more manageable are summarized in the box on the next page and described further in the next few pages. Use Exercise 5.1 to tailor these strategies to your own needs.

TAKING A LONG-TERM PERSPECTIVE

When Chang continued to confront Ming about how painful her affair had been for him, her guilt overwhelmed her and she responded with

> ## Strategies for Attending to Your Emotional Needs
>
> - Reminding yourself of long-term goals
> - Using self-talk to challenge fears or despair
> - Riding out difficult feelings until they pass
> - Venting feelings while away from your partner
> - Redirecting your thoughts or increasing positive experiences
> - Engaging in meditation, prayer, or other sources of inspiration

angry outbursts, blaming Chang for her affair. Chang would then withdraw into angry silence, unwilling to even consider his own role in their relationship. They became stuck in a destructive cycle of attacks and counterattacks that interfered with their recovery from the affair.

When your feelings in the moment seem overwhelming but your reactions to those feelings seem to make things worse, carefully consider your long-term goals for yourself and your relationship. If your long-term goal is to rebuild your relationship, then losing your temper and repeatedly lashing out at your partner won't help. If your long-term goal is to help your partner feel emotionally more secure, then walking away each time your partner expresses upset feelings is counterproductive. Tolerating distress and refraining from destructive reactions become easier when you remind yourself of your long-term individual and relationship goals.

USING HEALTHY SELF-TALK

Healthy "self-talk" means talking to yourself so you can stay on track and focused on what's helpful to you and your relationship. Self-talk can help you get through strong feelings in the moment: "Okay, this feels terrible right now. But that doesn't mean it's always going to feel this way. If I can try to get through this one day at a time, eventually things can get better." And it can help you assert personal control over your own behavior: "I'm not going to let that argument take over my whole life. There are still good things in my life, and I need to enjoy them."

Self-talk can also help you challenge false beliefs and other thoughts that may not be serving you well. Once a relationship starts to go sour, people often interpret a partner's behavior in the most negative possible way. But seeing your partner as purely evil or without any good qualities just makes things worse. Challenge your interpretations by asking yourself, "Why am I upset? Are there other possible explanations for what my partner just did or said that would be less upsetting?"

Unhealthy self-talk can sometimes *create or increase* negative emotions. For example, you may be telling yourself that this situation will never get better, or you may blame yourself for your partner's affair or believe the future is hopeless. Step back from your feelings and examine whether any self-talk may be contributing to them. For example, is there a difference between your partner's doing something really hurtful and being a horrible person? Did your own contributions to relationship problems in the past really make you responsible for your partner's affair? Are you likely to feel this miserable for the rest of your life? When you step back and challenge some of your negative thoughts, chances are you'll come up with a more balanced view of the situation that brings your emotions to a more bearable level.

"RIDING OUT" YOUR FEELINGS

Intensely painful feelings often feel like they'll never end. But as strong as these emotions may feel in the present moment, if you "ride out the wave," the feelings will often reach a peak and then diminish on their own. People sometimes deepen or prolong their distress by berating themselves for having their feelings in the first place. Instead, imagine these intense feelings as a wave and anticipate that they will eventually decline. The increased emotional distance can also allow you to think more clearly about what your feelings are and what triggered them.

> Ryan struggled to manage both his anger and anxiety when he and Dan argued. He would sometimes pursue the argument and escalate their conflict until one of them pushed or shoved the other. Once Ryan learned that emotions were like waves and that he could ride them out until they decreased to a more tolerable level on their own, he was able to stop his

*demands that Dan do something to make him feel better, which in turn
had been provoking even stronger arguments.*

Learning to ride out difficult feelings can also be helpful for involved partners, who sometimes struggle with waves of missing the outside person. If you've ended an affair and are committed to rebuilding your primary relationship but sometimes still have strong feelings for the outside person and urges to renew contact, redirecting your thoughts or activities elsewhere to ride out these feelings can be an effective way of dealing with your own emotional needs. We've worked with involved partners who have misinterpreted such feelings as an indication that a relationship with the outside person was "meant to be," only to regret responding to these feelings later on.

VENTING

Although at times you may be able to ride out intense emotions, at other times you may need strategies for "skimming" or "taking the edge off" your feelings to bring them down to a more manageable level. "Venting" is one way of making feelings more manageable. In Chapter 3 we described letters written for the sake of venting that are destroyed after being written without sending them to your partner. Another means of venting is to talk with someone you trust to hear your uncensored feelings. A close friend can serve as an outlet for venting, by phone or in person, but be sure you choose the appropriate person using guidelines we described in Chapter 4. And don't overdo it—even good friends can grow tired of long or frequent venting sessions. A trusted mental health or other helping professional might also be a good resource at these times.

GAINING DISTANCE

You can also gain some distance by using the time-out techniques discussed in Chapter 3 or by distracting yourself from thinking about the affair. Going for a walk, surfing the web or watching TV, or engaging in a hobby may provide just enough relief in the short run to allow you to manage your feelings and then address them more effectively either individually or with your partner. We're not suggesting that you avoid addressing problems, but there are times when you and your partner need to get away from them. Distracting yourself can be a healthy way to cope when problems feel overwhelming.

INCREASING POSITIVE EXPERIENCES

Healthy emotional self-care involves more than managing negative feelings—it also involves increasing positive experiences. When people are anxious or depressed, they're more likely to withdraw and stop pursuing pleasurable or rewarding activities. However, inactivity tends to increase depression and isolation, which makes you feel even less like doing anything pleasurable. This downward spiral is difficult to escape if you continue to do things only when you "feel like it." Instead, it's important that you commit to doing something good for yourself on a regular basis, even if it's just a relaxing bath at the end of the day, a weekly massage, or meeting one of your friends after work. Committing to pleasurable activities is critical to ensuring that you'll have the emotional reserves you need to get through this tough time and to treat the people around you well.

ENGAGING IN MEDITATION OR SPIRITUAL LIFE

During times of crisis many people draw on their spiritual life, while others find it helpful to deepen their spirituality if this part of their life has been lacking, perhaps reflecting on how they understand the world more broadly or reassessing their participation in their religious community. Attending to your spiritual needs may promote a feeling of inner strength or help in reflecting on broader or more complex questions, such as "What do I value the most in life?" "How do I reconcile what I value with what I've done?" "What do I believe about forgiveness or reconciliation?" or "How do I find meaning or purpose in this crisis?"

An individual's spirituality is a profoundly personal experience. If spirituality has been an important part of your life in the past, or if you believe that it might be helpful to you during this particularly difficult time, we encourage you to pursue your spiritual life in whatever ways may serve you best. Some people may renew their involvement in a local religious group. Others engage in meditation or prayer. You might find strength or inspiration in reading accounts of other persons' survival of traumatic experiences or triumphs over immense challenges. We don't presume to tell you *how* to attend to your spiritual needs. But we do encourage you to consider your spiritual life as one important way of caring for yourself.

Attending to Social Needs

Social support not only can help decrease emotional turmoil but also promotes physical health during times of stress. Close friends or family members can provide you with care and concern, help you talk through your feelings, reduce deep loneliness, and encourage you to take care of yourself both emotionally and physically.

Remember to be clear about what kind of support you want from which people. Maybe there are only one or two individuals you would want to talk with about the affair, but others whom you might tell that you and your partner have stopped going out together with other couples for the time being so they'll be more inclined to invite you to spend time together one-on-one. You might also find social support by spending more time in group functions related to your work, your children's school, or your neighborhood.

> Kelsey was sure her distress over Erik's betrayal was written all over her face. She withdrew from her regular book group and avoided her neighbors, but she soon noticed that her isolation was deepening her feelings of despair. To counteract this, she arranged a few lunches with close friends who were sensitive and supportive. Two of her friends invited her to a women's night out at an art gallery. The next day, her future didn't seem as bleak as it had the day before, and she vowed to make these outings regular events.

Attending to Physical Needs

Emotional and physical self-care go hand in hand—so make sure you're getting adequate sleep, nutrition, and exercise. Even if you believe you're managing these functions well for now, read through the physical self-care strategies discussed below and consider whether there are ways to implement these better, now or in the future.

SLEEP AND REST

Learn about and follow good sleep practices. Avoid taking naps or limit them to 20 minutes in the morning or early afternoon, so you will be sleepy at night. Also avoid caffeine, alcohol, or other mood-altering substances in large quantities or late in the day—all of which are likely to interfere with your sleep patterns. Try to get up and go to bed at the same times every day and develop a relaxing winding-down routine before bed. If you can't fall asleep after 20 minutes, instead of lying in bed worrying, get up and spend 20 minutes doing some quiet activity. Avoid watching TV because it's easy to get caught up in late-night talk shows or streaming options instead of falling asleep. After 20 minutes, go back to bed and try again. Avoid over-the-counter sleeping pills; they're likely to cause a rebound effect and continue your sleeping problems once you discontinue their use. If you're still unable to reclaim a nearly normal sleeping pattern after applying these strategies, consider discussing your sleep problems with your physician or a sleep specialist if your sleep problems have become severe.

NUTRITION

Healthy eating is literally one way to nurture yourself during this difficult time. If your blood sugar and protein levels drop too low, your ability to regulate your emotions also decreases, causing you to act impulsively and probably more intensely than you would if you were well rested and well fed. Taking time at regular intervals to eat some fruit, consume some protein, and provide your body with some form of complex carbohydrate should help you keep your emotions on a more even keel.

EXERCISE

You may feel too tired or too worn out by daily stressors or by the intense emotions you're feeling to even contemplate exercising. Or you may believe you can't afford to take the time away from your family or your other responsibilities to pursue it. *Our view is: You can't afford not to.* Regular, moderate exercise helps people reduce their feelings of anxiety and depression significantly; it also increases endorphins, the hormones released when we engage in pleasurable events such as sexual activity.

If exercise hasn't been part of your routine before, start with small goals—for example, taking a brisk walk three times a week. Schedule times for exercise when you're least likely to be distracted or interrupted, just as you would for other vital tasks. Variety in exercise routines (even walking in different directions around the block!) can help prevent boredom. Set modest goals and don't let a lapse of a day or two prevent you from starting up your routine again.

HEALTH

Physical illness and related health problems reduce your emotional resilience and decrease your ability to cope with individual and relationship challenges. If you've recently developed physical problems or have been putting off getting medical attention for an ongoing condition, make an appointment today. Taking time to visit your physician and complying with treatment will help you deal more effectively with your emotional difficulties in the long run.

Similarly, make healthy choices to limit alcohol, caffeine, and other nonprescription psychoactive substances not only because they can interfere with sleep as noted above but because they can make your existing mood problems worse. Caffeine and nicotine can increase emotional irritability. Alcohol has a tendency to suppress inhibitions and may make you more likely to say and do things you might regret. Although all of these substances may appear to offer short-term relief from painful feelings, in the long term they increase the likelihood of your continuing to feel emotionally drained or out of control.

Should I Seek Professional Help?

Aaliyah's initial shock and anger after discovering Khalil's affair gradually turned into endless numbness. Weeks went by, but she simply couldn't function at a good level. Some days she stayed at home in bed for hours at a time, staring at the wall. Her job began to suffer, and eventually her supervisor told her that, unless she managed her responsibilities better, she would be fired. Aaliyah needed to pull herself together, but she had no idea how.

When Should I Seek Professional Help Just for Me?

Although there's no simple answer to this question, a general guideline is to *pursue separate help for yourself if*:

- ▪ Your responses to the affair are so intense that they could result in serious harm to yourself or others.

- ▪ Your emotional distress continues over an extended period of time at a level that prevents individual or relationship recovery.

Additional signs that you might benefit from outside assistance include the following.

- ▪ *Severe or persistent depression:* Severe disruption of your sleep, eating, or other physical self-care that could lead to negative consequences for your health. Profound and unshakable feelings of hopelessness, worthlessness, or guilt. Nearly complete loss of interest in daily activities involving work, home, friends, or family on an ongoing basis.

- ▪ *Severe or persistent anxiety:* Overwhelming fear or worry that disrupts your ability to concentrate or think clearly. Acute physical arousal resulting in severe headaches, muscle tension, stomach upset, or chest pains. Recurrent episodes of panic or chronic dread.

- ▪ *Rage or physical aggression against others:* Uncontrolled verbal or physical aggression directed toward your partner, the outside affair person, or others. Acts of retaliation against your partner that you later regret, such as destruction of property. Sudden outbursts of anger toward persons uninvolved in the affair, such as your children or coworkers.

- ▪ *Behaviors harmful to yourself:* Excessive use of alcohol or other substances to influence your mood, spending sprees that create financial hardship, or having an affair of your own as a way of "getting even." Harming yourself physically is a major warning sign calling for assistance.

- ▪ *Inability to reach critical decisions:* Inability to reach decisions for yourself about how to manage this crisis in the short term—such as how to confront your partner or the outside affair person or whether to continue living together. Or inability to approach longer-term decisions—for example, whether to commit to working on your relationship or moving on separately.

If one or more of these descriptions apply to you, it's important to get separate help for yourself. You might also decide to seek outside assistance even if your difficulties don't appear as severe as those described above. Getting outside help isn't weak or self-indulgent; it's about becoming healthy again for yourself and for the sake of those persons you care about and who care about you. Among the benefits that outside professionals may provide are expertise in dealing with relationship problems, ability to offer specific resources such as medication, greater capacity to remain objective, and commitment to confidentiality. Exercise 5.2 can help you decide whether and how to seek professional help. Here are some options regarding helping professionals you might consider.

How Can I Find Help—Either for Myself or for Both of Us Together?

Mental health professionals who provide counseling have many different backgrounds, levels of training, and areas of expertise. Licensed psychologists typically have a doctoral degree (PhD or PsyD) and at least five years of training beyond college in working with people experiencing emotional or behavioral problems. Social workers are usually licensed with a master's degree (MSW) and have two to three years of training beyond college. Most states also have licensed marital and family therapists with a master's degree (MA or MS) and may certify or license a separate group of professional counselors at the master's degree level. Psychiatrists first receive their training in medicine as physicians (MD or DO) and then pursue a two- to three-year specialized residency in psychiatry.

In addition to these differences in background, professional counselors differ widely in their approaches to individual and relationship problems. Some have extensive training and experience in treating individuals but little or none in working with couples or families. Some may focus primarily on your communication and current ways of behaving, while others might examine relationship patterns in the family you grew up with or underlying issues outside your immediate awareness that contribute to current difficulties.

If you're currently involved in a religious organization or other organization with leaders you respect, consider requesting counseling from someone in that organization if they are properly trained. They may also facilitate your spiritual life or suggest books that integrate spiritual with individual or relationship needs.

With all these options, how can you make an informed decision about where to get help? One approach is to seek recommendations from individuals in related professions. For example, your family physician may know of professional counselors with special expertise in helping people deal with relationship problems. If you live in a community with a college or university, there may be a university-affiliated clinic that offers individual or couple counseling. You may also know of a friend or family member who pursued professional counseling and can suggest someone to see or to call for a recommendation. If all else fails, search the web for listings of mental health professionals in your area and carefully review their backgrounds and areas of expertise; then schedule an initial consultation for yourself or for you and your partner together with a counselor who appears to be a potential resource. If you or your partner doesn't feel that the counselor is a good match after an initial meeting, ask for recommendations for alternative professionals in your area.

Complete both of the following exercises and encourage your partner to do the same. After completing these exercises, you're ready to move on to the next stage of recovery to work on understanding how this affair came about.

EXERCISES

EXERCISE 5.1 Attending to Your Emotional Needs

Review the guidelines in this chapter for taking care of your emotional needs and consider which strategies might work best for you. Be sure to include at least one strategy for managing negative feelings and one for increasing positive experiences. After one week if either strategy hasn't worked as well as you had hoped, consider what you could do to implement that strategy more effectively or what alternative strategies you might use.

Decide on Strategies for Managing Your Intense Negative Feelings

For example:

> "When I feel as though I'm about to explode from thinking about the affair, I'm going to pursue a separate activity to distract myself and get some relief. If that doesn't work, I'll write myself a letter as a way to 'unload' and will then tear it up."

Outline Specific Steps for Increasing Your Positive Experiences

For example:

> "I'm going to take 30 minutes each evening to do something for myself—whether it's going for a walk, meditating, or refinishing the bookcase."

EXERCISE 5.2 Deciding Whether to Seek Professional Help

Consider the potential benefits of getting outside help, either for you individually or for both of you together. If you're not sure how to identify possible resources, identify who might be able to offer a reliable referral. For example:

> "I'd prefer that my partner and I get some counseling together to help us manage our conflict better and reach some important decisions as a couple. I'll call our family doctor to see whom she would recommend. If my partner won't join me in these efforts, I'll pursue individual counseling for myself."

PART II

How Did
This Happen?

6

Was Our Relationship to Blame?

"It's time to put it behind us and move on," Trevor said firmly. "I know I screwed up, and I won't do it again. But now we need to focus on us and our future, not on the past." Arianna wanted nothing more than to move on. But to Trevor, moving on meant no longer discussing the affair. Arianna, however, kept thinking about the affair, no matter how hard she tried not to. How could he have done this? Had something been missing in their relationship? If so, could she count on Trevor to be faithful the next time they went through a difficult time? Until she was certain that both of them understood how and why his affair had occurred, Arianna couldn't trust that it wouldn't eventually happen again. She couldn't move on.

If you've worked successfully through the previous chapters—whether with your partner or largely on your own—your life may be feeling less chaotic or under better control. Restoring some of your daily routines, decreasing angry exchanges or some of the emotional distance between you, and taking care of yourselves can bring considerable relief to both of you at this time.

So why stir everything up? Why ask why? Why did the affair happen? How could you or your partner have done this? What went wrong? The reasons for asking why are simple, even if the implications of asking why are complex:

■ If you're the injured partner, you need to learn as much as you can about why this affair happened to restore the emotional security essential to trust and intimacy.

■ If you're the partner who had the affair, you need to explore why this affair happened *because it's what your partner needs*. And it could benefit you as well, because you need to understand your own behavior and decisions, if only to make sure you don't make the same mistake again.

Exploring how the affair came about is necessary to restoring the injured partner's sense of emotional security; it's the only way to get the injured party back on solid enough ground to even consider whether a relationship of trust and intimacy can be rebuilt. If you're the involved partner, there are also direct benefits for you such as understanding yourself better and making sure you're less likely to be tempted by infidelity or other kinds of deceit again.

In exploring how the affair came about, it's important to distinguish between *reasons* and *excuses*—and between *understanding* and *agreement*. If you're the injured person, no number of reasons will excuse your partner's affair. If you're the partner involved in the affair, you may not be asking to be excused. We want both of you to understand why the affair has occurred but not to agree with a partner's decision to have an affair. Understanding requires looking at the big picture—or what we call the context—for the affair. It involves examining all the factors that contributed to an increased risk, or vulnerability, that this affair would occur. None of these factors—individually or collectively—*caused* this affair. Ultimately, responsibility for having an affair rests with the person who chose to engage in the affair, consciously or not, in response to whatever created the risk or vulnerability. We repeat: *If you had an affair, you're responsible for your own behavior.* At the same time, we want to help both of you understand the factors that might have made you vulnerable to making the decisions you made.

In these next four chapters, we'll guide you through a process of systematically exploring a broad range of potential factors that may have contributed to your relationship's vulnerability to an affair. This exploration requires stirring things up and tolerating more discomfort in the short run. There may be issues in your relationship or aspects of each of you that are difficult to acknowledge and perhaps painful to discuss. But our decades of collective experience with couples struggling after an affair have shown that *coming to a fuller understanding of why an affair occurred is simultaneously the most difficult and also the most important stage of recovery.* Couples who commit to this process use the crisis of an affair to identify changes they could make to restore emotional security and joy between them. Many relationships end up even stronger than they were before the affair.

Couples who avoid this process will instead experience two significant risks:

1. After an initial period of stability—which may last a few months or even a few years—the doubts and unanswered questions of how the affair happened often resurface. At that point, the issues are much more difficult to explore, and the relationship ends in confusion and bitterness.

2. Alternatively, the unanswered questions are buried and pushed out of awareness but continue to fester beneath the surface. Couples following this path may stay together—but emotional intimacy, joy, and passion can fade away. Detachment takes over.

How Much Do We Need to Know?

A lot! An affair calls everything into question. And from the injured partner's perspective, beneath any unturned stone lurks another danger—the chance that whatever led to this affair could lead to another. Each of these next four chapters focuses on a different set of factors that may have increased the vulnerability of your relationship to an affair. You've probably already thought about many of them, but here is a preview.

WHAT WAS HAPPENING IN YOUR RELATIONSHIP

Affairs don't occur because of a bad relationship. There are plenty of troubled relationships that don't end up experiencing an affair, and affairs can occur even when the person having the affair reports having been satisfied and in love with their partner. We'll never suggest that you blame your relationship for the affair. However, it's also important that both of you take a hard look at what was going on in your relationship that might have made it more vulnerable or susceptible to one partner deciding to have an affair. Later in this chapter we'll help you explore the following:

- Levels and sources of conflict
- Emotional connectedness
- Physical intimacy
- Relationship roles and expectations

WHAT WAS HAPPENING AROUND AND OUTSIDE OF YOUR RELATIONSHIP?

Maintaining a strong relationship requires hard work. That work becomes even more difficult when either (1) other people actively undermine your efforts to care for one another and remain faithful or (2) you fail to receive adequate support and encouragement for your relationship. In Chapter 7, we'll help you consider each of the following:

- Intrusions and distractions
- Outside stressors
- Temptations
- Supports

WHAT THE INVOLVED PARTNER BROUGHT TO THE AFFAIR

As the injured party, you need to figure out why your partner got involved in an affair—regardless of whatever else was going on between or around you. Viewing your partner only in negative ways—as fundamentally defective and without moral fiber—may fit with the hurt and anger you feel but won't help to restore feelings of closeness or security. You need to be able to view your partner using a wide-angle lens—seeing strengths as well as shortcomings, virtues as well as flaws—to reach good decisions about how to move on.

If you're the involved partner, it's also important that you carefully examine what aspects of yourself contributed to your having an affair. Understanding yourself at a deeper level, including your own personal needs or conflicts, will help you ensure that this doesn't happen to you again, whether you stay in this relationship or not. *Promising never to have another affair isn't enough.* Understanding how you got there and what you need to change will help you keep any promises you make to yourself or someone else.

Chapter 8 will help you both gain this fuller understanding by examining the following areas:

- Personal qualities increasing your vulnerability to an affair
- Beliefs about affairs and commitment to your relationship
- Barriers to moving on

WHAT THE INJURED PARTNER CONTRIBUTED TO THE CONTEXT FOR THE AFFAIR

Remember that no one causes their partner to have an affair. The questions we encourage injured partners to explore are these: "If my relationship became vulnerable to an affair because of conflict, emotional disconnection, outside commitments, or any other reason, could I have contributed to that vulnerability? What could I have done differently?" Answers to these questions empower you to take steps to address any ways in which you may have contributed to your relationship's increased vulnerability so you'll be better protected in the future. You both are responsible for how you behave in your relationship; your partner is responsible for the affair.

If you're the involved partner, only *you* know how your feelings about your relationship and your partner may have contributed to the context for your affair. Your partner needs your perspectives as well as your encouragement to explore their own role in your relationship and steps to make it stronger and more secure, keeping in mind that your partner is not responsible for your affair.

If you're the injured partner, in Chapter 9 we'll guide you in examining possible contributing factors similar to those we've already identified for the involved partner, as well as others unique to the injured partner:

- Feelings about yourself
- Contributions to your relationship
- Responses to personal injuries

Take It a Step at a Time

If you rush through this next stage too quickly, you won't examine some contributing factors closely or deeply enough; then you'll either (1) continue to feel uneasy or frustrated with lingering issues that haven't been addressed or (2) settle on an incomplete picture that leaves your relationship more vulnerable later on. Tailor the process to the emotional resources and time you can each commit, as well as to your ability to keep your interactions constructive. Also, be sure to spend time together each week *not* discussing the affair but, instead, restoring positive ways of being together that you enjoyed in the past. Caring for yourselves and your relationship will give you the hope and the emotional energy essential to getting through this next stage.

One approach for working through these next four chapters is to set aside one or two times a week, for about 30 minutes on each occasion, to discuss what you've read or share your responses to an exercise. At the end of each interaction with your partner, try to agree on when you'll get together next and what you'll read or work on before then. Avoid getting stuck for too long on any one question. You can always come back to an earlier issue, and the work you've done between times may help you reconsider previous questions from a different perspective.

Whether you're the injured partner or the involved partner, if you're ready to engage this next stage and explore contributing factors but your partner remains reluctant to join in this process, you have a few options:

- You can talk through the reasons for your partner's reluctance so that you can address them and then work together collaboratively. Share your concerns about not examining how the affair came about and the potential advantages of doing so. Express your confidence in your ability to do this, for example, by pointing to progress you've made so far or to earlier times in your relationship when you were able to work together to address problems. Use Exercise 6.1 to help you in this discussion.

- You can do most of the work by yourself but then try to share the results of your efforts with your partner to invite a response. For example, perhaps your partner isn't ready to read through the chapters and exercises with you but is willing to have discussions with you based on your own reading. *Any* constructive work together is better than none, so try to find an initial compromise that will allow you to share your thoughts and feelings as you work through the next few chapters.

That said, if you're the reluctant partner, understand that encouraging your partner to share their efforts without you also working on these issues will eventually fall short. Your relationship won't recover fully until you're each convinced of the other person's commitment to doing whatever it takes to move forward. Doing this work is a critical signal that you're willing to repair the damage to the relationship from your affair.

■ You can pursue the process completely separately from your partner and then use what you've learned to work at change by yourself—either for the sake of staying in this relationship or to be better informed about yourself and relationships generally if you decide to end this one.

Was Our Relationship the Cause?

Abby and Colin each believed they had "the perfect relationship." The first few years as a couple were happy, and they built a successful business together. Life was good. Eventually they decided to begin a family of their own. Abby turned their business over to Colin while she stayed home to care for their two sons, who arrived over the next three years. Pleased at first with these decisions, neither was prepared for their new roles.

Abby had few friends of her own and turned increasingly to Colin for comfort and relief from the children when he came home in the evenings. The more she needed Colin, however, the less available he appeared to be. His hours at work grew longer, and his patience at home seemed to grow shorter. Colin struggled too. This wasn't what he had expected fatherhood to feel like. He was uncomfortable holding the boys when they cried and felt impatient when they constantly demanded his attention. Abby couldn't appreciate his difficulties with the boys and frequently seemed angry at him for reasons he didn't understand.

When their sons reached ages two and four, Abby and Colin placed them in daycare two afternoons each week so that Abby could take a business class at their community college. There she found other adults her age who were juggling multiple challenges of work, family, and school. One in particular, Ben, was very friendly to Abby and seemed especially understanding. Ben was divorced, and Abby admired his devotion to his daughter from that marriage. Increasingly Abby felt drawn to Ben, who empathized with her loneliness and eventually disclosed his own increasing emotional and physical attraction to her.

Following a week when she and Colin had argued almost constantly and slept in separate rooms, Abby visited Ben at his apartment. She felt abandoned by Colin. She knew having an affair would be wrong, but her longing to be held and comforted overcame her. She and Ben ended up in bed together that afternoon, then twice more in the following week.

Over the next two months Abby wrestled with guilt and confusion about the dual life she was leading. She broke off her relationship with Ben, but two weeks later disclosed her affair to Colin and asked that they live separately for a while to give them space to reach a decision about their relationship. Both of them felt hurt, angry, and confused. Colin felt devastated and utterly betrayed by Abby; he hadn't done anything to deserve this. But he also didn't want to lose Abby. He and Abby agreed they needed help to reach a decision about what to do next. In couple therapy they were able to reach some short-term decisions about how to interact with each other and around their children. Once they got through their initial crisis, they began to consider all that had gone wrong. How did this happen? They once had a wonderful relationship. How did it come tumbling apart?

When your partner has had an affair, you may ask yourself, "Was our relationship to blame?" The answer to that is a firm "No." Responsibility rests with the person who chose to have an affair. But you *should* consider how your relationship became vulnerable to an affair. Were important qualities missing? Were there ways you two could have made your relationship stronger? As you look back, you may be able to identify several aspects of your relationship that weren't as healthy or satisfying as either one of you might have liked. The goal in thinking about how you got here isn't to lay blame—it's to figure out how you could make your relationship more secure now.

Right now, your mind may be reeling with negative thoughts about your partner: they had the affair because they're unloving, untrustworthy, or can't commit. You're absolutely right to want to know how your partner could have done such a hurtful thing. But remember that this is the same person you fell in love with and expected to spend a good part of your life with; it's likely that the same good qualities you fell in love with are still there now. To make sense of how this person you've loved could have done such a hurtful thing, it's important to consider how your relationship might have influenced your partner's decision to have an affair.

Involved partners need to gain the same insight. Few, if any, pledged a vow of commitment while also *intending* to be unfaithful. Many that we've counseled, in fact, describe being bewildered by how they could have ended up on this path. To make sense of their own behavior, involved partners as well as injured partners need to examine not only aspects of themselves individually but also risk factors outside of themselves, including the relationship itself.

In the remainder of this chapter, we'll offer a process for doing just that. We'll guide you in examining various aspects of your relationship in the three to four months prior to the beginning of the affair and then also viewing your relationship from a broader perspective—including initial sources of attraction to each other and patterns of interacting since early in your relationship. Finally, we'll help you address one of the most important questions you'll face: *Given everything you and your partner can learn about potential vulnerabilities in your relationship, what would it take to make your relationship more secure now?*

As you go through this chapter, remember that you're looking at only one part of the puzzle. Try to avoid quickly settling on any one conclusion about how this affair came about, because premature conclusions based on a limited view can get in the way of examining the bigger picture. Chapters 7 through 9 will help you examine other aspects of your life as a couple and as individuals. Later, you can step back and put all these pieces together into a coherent story. In addition, try to distinguish among different time periods in your relationship—for example, during courtship, the first few years as a couple, and the last few years. As hard as this may sound, try not to let your struggles since the affair determine how you view your relationship in earlier years. Understanding both the good and not-so-good periods can help you consider your relationship when it's at its best and begin to identify factors that might have contributed or still contribute to relationship difficulties.

What Was Our Relationship Like
Before the Affair?

The following questions address a variety of issues that can expose relationships to distress and may have made your relationship more vulnerable. Although a struggling relationship doesn't *cause* an affair, experiencing lots of conflict or being unfulfilled in a relationship can be one reason some partners turn to someone else. These questions don't cover all possible concerns but can help to get you started in this process.

How Well Did We Deal with Disagreements?

One of the most common complaints among distressed couples involves difficulties managing conflict. The specific form that such conflict takes can vary a lot. For some couples, even minor disagreements or differences escalate into major arguments; a pattern of intense conflict with few agreements leads to a backlog of unresolved differences that drives partners apart emotionally and physically. For other couples, differences between partners are rarely acknowledged or openly discussed; however, either partner may feel frustrated or resentful when issues important to that person aren't recognized or resolved. Still other couples describe a pattern of frequent bickering that erodes their sense of closeness or liking for one another; tensions may occasionally erupt into major conflicts, or they're evident from minor but frequent skirmishes with no predictable pattern.

Any one of these patterns for dealing with disagreements can increase a couple's distress and vulnerability to an affair. To examine how well you and your partner dealt with differences before the affair, consider the *overall level of conflict* there was in your relationship as well as the *various areas that led to conflict*. Also, it's important to understand the ways that you used to manage the conflict and how successful those approaches were. We'll raise initial questions for you to consider here. Then, use Exercise 6.2 to develop a clearer picture of how the two of you have managed conflict in the past and how you could do it more effectively in the future.

LEVELS OF CONFLICT

It's not the fact that you two disagree that matters—virtually all couples have disagreements—but it's how you manage the disagreements. The frequency, intensity, and duration of conflicts can increase your relationship's vulnerability to an affair. How *often* did you and your partner argue in the few months before the affair? Had arguments become more common, perhaps reflecting a growing frustration with your relationship? Or had arguments become less frequent, perhaps because one of you had given up on resolving differences over important issues?

How *intense* were the conflicts? Did they typically involve minor bickering or major arguments that escalated out of proportion? Did they lead either one of you to threaten or consider ending your relationship? And how *long* did your arguments last—a few minutes, a few hours, or days? Following a disagreement, how long did it typically take you to reconnect either by resolving the difference or by accepting it and moving on? Did you and your partner frequently have different "recovery times"? How did you approach each other after a conflict to reconnect or try to make things right and move on?

Were there times when you were able to address differences effectively—perhaps by using some of the communication skills described in Chapter 3? What distinguished times the two of you managed conflict better from the times you fell short?

SOURCES OF CONFLICT

If you ask someone what topics couples argue about most, common answers might be sex, money, children, and in-laws. Many times, however, the picture is more complicated. Conflicts about children, for example, may involve differences in fundamental values, expectations regarding partners' respective child-rearing responsibilities, or beliefs about best methods of discipline. If you and your partner have trouble pinpointing the primary sources of conflict in your relationship or disagree on what might help to eliminate or reduce the conflict, step back and ask yourself, "What else might be going on here that we're not recognizing?"

We'll describe common sources of relationship conflict (listed in the box on this page) below. As you think about each of these areas, begin thinking about strengths in your relationship as well as problems.

Conflicts in Specific Areas. Consider where you and your partner have experienced frequent or intense conflict—for example, about finances, the children, your sexual relationship, how to spend your leisure time, or how to divide responsibilities in the home. Try to rank-order these into the "hottest" two or three conflict areas—the ones that really get in your way and feel the worst. How have conflicts in these areas changed over the years? Also try to identify times when you managed differences in these areas with less conflict. What did you and your partner do differently at those times that seemed to work better?

Conflicts Related to Boundaries. Boundaries are essential for defining what couples share versus keep separate from each other in their individual lives and what they keep separate as a couple from others. Partners can differ in where they think these boundaries should go. For example, partners might differ in terms of what information they believe is appropriate to share with other people. That is, one person might want to talk with parents about the couple's finances or their plans to have a child soon, but

---

Common sources of relationship conflict include the following:

- Conflicts in specific areas—for example, finances, children, or household responsibilities
- Disagreements about boundaries—for example, time spent separately or together with friends or family
- Division of shared resources—such as money, time, or physical space in the home
- Imbalances of opportunities or responsibilities—including career decisions
- Differences in preferences or values—for example, sleep schedules or political views
- Differences in personal style—such as emotional expressiveness or activity level

the other partner might consider these issues "private" and definitely not a topic of conversation with parents. More directly related to affairs, the two partners might also have different beliefs about what's acceptable to share both physically and emotionally with another person (friend, coworker, acquaintance) outside of their relationship. These struggles around boundaries can have a strong impact on how close a partner feels with people outside of the couple's relationship.

> Bryce was Shawn's first and only committed romantic partner, but Shawn knew that Bryce had been in several prior romantic relationships. When they moved in together, Shawn assumed that Bryce would end all communication with his previous partners, even the ones that had faded into just friendship. Bryce had different expectations. He was devoted to Shawn but didn't see the need to sever his close friendships with partners from the past—he still valued their opinions when he needed advice and didn't see any issue with having them as an integral part of his daily life. Bryce and Shawn's brief discussions on this issue never ended well, and they increasingly avoided the topic. When Shawn learned from a mutual friend that Bryce was continuing to meet a previous partner for lunch once a week, he felt deceived and betrayed. When Shawn brought it up, Bryce felt unfairly attacked because the two of them had never reached an explicit agreement about the boundaries of their relationship.

Partners might also differ in the types of boundaries they want between the two of them as individuals; for example, one partner may want times alone with personal friends, whereas the other partner wants both partners to be included anytime there's interaction with friends. Have differences in your preferences concerning various types of boundaries contributed to conflicts in your relationship in the past? Do you and your partner agree on how much time to spend apart or with others? Do you agree on what kinds of communication and interactions to keep for just the two of you?

Conflicts Related to Shared Resources. Some couples have difficulty defining "yours, mine, or ours" in different areas, from money and material objects to time and physical space in the home. Even when they seem trivial, such conflicts can trigger strong feelings—such as how to divide the space in a cramped clothes closet. What strategies have you and your partner used to promote feelings of fairness for both of you?

Conflicts Related to Opportunities and Responsibilities. Partners sometimes struggle with how to balance their individual opportunities and responsibilities in their relationship. For example, pursuing a career outside the home may be viewed by one partner as an *opportunity* for individual growth but by the other as a *responsibility* to provide financially for the family. When couples maintain a "team identity," each partner can contribute at different times or in different ways that feel fair and mutually encouraging. In what ways have you and your partner struggled to maintain a "team identity" in your own relationship where you both feel good about your relative contributions?

Conflicts Related to Different Preferences and Values. Relationship conflict can result from differences in preferences or core values. By preferences we mean likes and dislikes (going to the movies versus watching shows at home, for example), and such differences can often be tolerated or negotiated to find a middle ground. However, even small differences in preferences can become burdensome if it seems that almost everything has to be negotiated—different food preferences, sleep schedules, vacation styles, and the like.

Core values, by comparison, involve what someone holds as dear or deeply important and may include spiritual or moral principles. Understandably, differences in core values can be more difficult to resolve because individuals don't easily give up or shift their core ideals. For example, not being totally truthful when filing taxes might seem fine to one partner but be viewed by the other partner as immoral or unacceptable. Furthermore, some couples have difficulty resolving differences because they label almost everything as a core value and nothing as a mere preference. When too many differences are framed as critical issues involving core values, partners can find themselves deeply stuck in opposing views and unwilling to budge toward a middle position. How often in the past have you and your partner gotten stuck because you could not resolve minor or moderate differences in preferences, struggled around a core value, or got caught in a stalemate because preferences were handled as though they involved conflicting core values?

Conflicts Related to Differences in Personal Style. Couples can struggle with individual differences in personal style—levels of emotional expressiveness, activity level, decision-making style, and so on. Early on in relationships, such differences can feel complementary or help to balance each other out (as in "opposites attract"), but later they can become polarizing and feel incompatible. For example, initially one partner's free-spirited style might seem exciting and colorful to the other partner, but years later that style can also seem disorganized and frustrating. To what extent have conflicts between you and your partner resulted from differences that seem to be part of your core personalities—for example, who prefers to be in charge, how much activity you each like, or whether you favor discussing feelings versus solving problems? Instead of undermining your relationship, how could you use such differences to strengthen it?

> Uri and Olivia argued constantly about planning and being on time. Olivia liked to look ahead and plan in detail to make things run smoothly. Uri was more laid back and liked to approach life more spontaneously. Not surprisingly, they also viewed time differently. Olivia preferred to arrive early for any activity and build in a cushion in case something went wrong. Uri's view was "It's no big deal if you're a little late—just relax." Over time, they recognized that neither of them would change their basic attitudes toward planning and time, but they could decide together which occasions merited more planning and timeliness versus those when they could be more relaxed and spontaneous.

DIFFICULTIES IN MANAGING CONFLICT

Because some level of conflict is inevitable in intimate relationships, couples need strategies for identifying differences, preventing conflicts from escalating into destructive arguments, and reaching decisions together in a way that resolves differences or makes them more tolerable. Ineffective strategies for managing conflict may stem from the following:

- Under- or overcontrol of feelings
- Differences in emotional and cognitive style
- Differences in timing
- Efforts to win

Under- or Overcontrol of Emotions. Some couples run "too hot." Every disagreement or frustration—no matter how small—demands discussion about "what's wrong" and ignores "what's right" in the relationship. By contrast, some relationships run "too cold." Partners pursue peace and comfort by avoiding difficult but important discussions, which can lead to an increasing sense of being distant from each other. Before the affair, how much balance did you achieve in managing conflict, discussing important relationship issues but letting go of minor irritations or annoyances?

Differences in Emotional and Cognitive Style. There's some evidence that women are typically brought up to discuss feelings as a way of promoting closeness, whereas men are often encouraged to treat conflicts as problems to be solved through dispassionate analysis. Neither approach is inherently better than the other; actually, good solutions often take both emotion and logic into account. It's important for partners to understand differences in their styles and learn how to accommodate both when dealing with relationship conflicts. These differences in style in focusing on emotions versus logic can be one reason that couples at times can feel "out of sync" when discussing differences. Has either of you viewed the other as too focused on feelings or logic in approaching problems?

Differences in Timing. Some people feel a strong need to resolve tensions right away, while others need time apart to gain perspective and better control over their feelings before coming together to discuss the issue. When one partner seeks immediate resolution and the other needs time to calm down emotionally or think things through individually before talking together, efforts to resolve conflict together may not be productive. To what extent have you and your partner experienced different preferences in this regard?

> When dealing with differences of opinion, Ethan tended to become heated but would then cool down and look for common ground. Haley sometimes felt wounded by Ethan's comments; she continued to feel hurt long after he had already cooled down and wasn't yet ready to resume discussion—a response that Ethan viewed as unforgiving and punitive.

Their discussions improved when Ethan exercised better control over how he expressed his opinions and when Haley learned to tolerate some of her own discomfort with conflict.

Efforts to Win. When efforts to resolve differences have less to do with collaboration and more to do with who's "right," the relationship ends up losing. *Neither partner can win an argument without the other losing.* Strategies for resolving conflict work best when both partners shift from a focus on what *they* want to a focus on what their *relationship* needs. How often have efforts to resolve conflicts gotten stuck because they felt like a win–lose struggle? Or you both make a strong argument for what you each prefer, and then you hit a stalemate because neither of you wants to back down? What would it take from *you* to promote a stronger sense of team-work and collaboration?

Most of the topics we've raised so far involve difficulties dealing with complex or negative aspects of the relationship in unproductive ways. In addition, it's important that couples experience positive aspects of their relationships. Too few positive experiences can lead to a less rewarding relationship as well—something we'll help you consider next.

How Emotionally Connected Did We Feel?

Most likely you and your partner were attracted to each other because you enjoyed each other's company. There was something about being with your partner that simply felt good. It may be because you shared similar inter-ests and had fun together. Or perhaps you found your partner easy to talk with and able to understand your feelings. Perhaps your partner was espe-cially supportive through a difficult time. Any one of these experiences helps to promote a feeling of being emotionally connected.

Partners can feel emotionally disconnected even when they're not experiencing conflict; in those instances, the relationship can feel some-what "flat." In considering how your relationship became vulnerable to an affair, it's important to consider how the two of you may have drifted apart. We list some ways of becoming emotionally disconnected in the box on the next page; below we describe strategies couples use to promote feelings of emotional closeness in their relationships.

Ways of becoming emotionally disconnected include the following:

- Not working together as a team to accomplish common tasks

- Difficulty in sharing emotional experiences or feeling understood

- Not sharing visions or dreams for the future

- Not setting aside enough time to play or have fun together

SHARING EXPERIENCES

Partners feel closer to each other when they arrange times to work side by side for the sole purpose of spending time together. For example, some couples make it a point to prepare meals or work in the yard together; others read stories to their children or run errands together. Couples also pursue connection by talking with each other about everyday experiences or sitting close together on the couch while watching TV.

On a deeper level, couples often feel most emotionally connected when one partner shares feelings of hurt, disappointment, or other vulnerable emotions and the other listens in a caring and supportive way. Partners' abilities to share deep feelings, to have these feelings heard and understood, and to experience a tender caring for each other form a very important part of many intimate relationships. In thinking about your own relationship, how well did both you and your partner demonstrate your interest and concern for each other before the affair? Did you invite each other to share your deepest thoughts and feelings, and did you genuinely listen to each other?

SHARING VISIONS

Partners feel emotionally connected when they share a common vision. The vision may be as simple as how to plan new landscaping in the yard. Or it may be as complicated as how to pursue a value-driven or meaningful life together.

It's easy for couples to lose a sense of shared vision. We've listened to many couples describe how earlier in their courtship they used to sit for hours talking about their visions of how their family life would be:

how many children to have and what to name them, places they'd travel to together, or what they wanted to contribute to the world. But years later the experience of sharing visions somehow got lost. Sometimes their dreams suffered under the weight of current disappointments, or the reality of today's demands offered little opportunity for dreaming about tomorrow.

Sharing a vision for the future can be as important as sharing feelings from today's events. Right now, the future of your relationship may feel too uncertain to experience a shared vision. But try to recall the three to four months prior to the affair. How often did you and your partner share dreams for your future together?

SHARING PLAY AND FUN

Sharing laughter, playing games, pursuing common activities, and simply relaxing together are some of the ways that partners connect. Research shows that couples who spend significant amounts of time together in common activities other than work also report more satisfaction with their relationship. Stated simply, *couples who play together are more likely to stay together.*

There are two general kinds of pleasurable activities that couples use for reconnecting. "Parallel" activities such as watching a movie, reading quietly in the same room, or attending an event together can be a way of sharing time and space when tensions between partners may make it more difficult to interact without getting into conflict or hurtful discussions. By contrast, "joint" activities such as preparing a romantic dinner together, going for a leisurely stroll, pursuing a hobby together, or other activities that call for direct interaction often work best when tensions between partners are fewer or can be put aside.

Some couples allow their play time to suffer in response to such demands as child rearing, responsibilities at work, or commitments to various organizations in their community. Before the affair, how well did the two of you preserve time to play together? When setting aside time for play, were you careful not to allow discussions about relationship problems to intrude? When previous ways of being together were no longer possible or lost their appeal, did you develop new ways of connecting through leisure time together? Use Exercise 6.3 to identify steps for restoring or creating more emotional closeness between the two of you.

How Physically Intimate Were We?

Just like emotional closeness, physical intimacy occurs on different levels. For many couples, touching and holding one another are just as important as sexual intimacy. The ways that couples can become physically disconnected are discussed below (and listed in the box below), along with strategies for promoting physical closeness.

NONSEXUAL INTIMACY

In considering the quality of physical intimacy between you and your partner prior to the affair, it may be useful to think first about physical closeness other than sexual exchanges. How often did you touch one another in caring but nonsexual ways? For example, did you usually hold hands when sitting together at a movie or ball game? Did you offer gentle or reassuring touches as you passed each other in the hallway or kitchen? How often did you touch or hold each other in bed when not making love?

Individuals vary in how comfortable they are with physical touch and how much they desire touching in nonsexual ways. How important is it to you and your partner to be physically close in nonsexual ways? How do you each express your need for such closeness or respond to your partner's needs? If you and your partner differ in these ways, how have you tried to find some middle ground? How physically affectionate were you around the time of the affair?

Ways of becoming physically disconnected include the following:

- Insufficient touches, hugs, or other nonsexual forms of physical closeness
- Differences in levels of sexual desire
- Low frequency of sexual intimacy
- Dissatisfaction with the quality of sexual intimacy
- Difficulties talking about sex
- Barriers to sexual intimacy

SEXUAL INTIMACY

For many couples, sexual intimacy is closely tied to how emotionally connected the partners feel—with sexual intimacy occurring more often when partners feel emotionally close, or emotional closeness following from sexual intimacy, or both. Other individuals or couples are able to maintain a satisfying sex life even when they're not getting along in other ways. Regardless, when sexual intimacy does decline or breaks down, partners' responses can include hurt or disappointment, confusion, or emotional and physical withdrawal.

> Raini enjoyed sexual interactions with Dyani and was almost always "in the mood." Dyani enjoyed sex with Raini, too, but after she was promoted at work, increased work stress affected her sex drive. In general, she also preferred relaxed and longer lovemaking—even if less often— to the frequent but sometimes quicker sex that Raini seemed comfortable with. Dyani didn't like disappointing Raini, and similarly he didn't like the idea of pressuring her. After a while they both found it easier to avoid dealing with differences around sex, and their lovemaking became less and less frequent. Neither felt happy about the situation, but they just couldn't seem to find ways of discussing it to make it better.

Differences in Sexual Desire and Low Frequency of Sexual Exchanges. It's not unusual for partners to differ in their overall desire for sexual intimacy or to differ at any given time. About 15% of men and 25% of women report that their disinterest in sex is a problem for them or their relationship. For many couples, sexual intimacy is particularly rewarding when both partners view it as an important part of their relationship, feel free to express their sexual desire, and assume some share of responsibility for initiating and responding to requests for sex. Feelings of guilt, pressure, or blame detract from enjoyment of sexual experiences. So do feelings of hurt, resentment, or overall unhappiness with the relationship.

Couples vary widely in how often they have sex, and there are some overall trends that are common as couples age. Couples in their 20s tend to engage in sexual interactions more frequently than couples in their 50s, but there are wide variations within age ranges. When sex occurs so infrequently that it feels like it isn't a part of their routine relationship, partners can begin to feel self-conscious or anxious about their sexual intimacy.

Sometimes this concern can even trigger a pattern of avoiding affection such as physical touch, hugs, or kissing out of concern that it might lead to a more explicit focus on sex. This pattern of avoidance can then feed more anxiety, which in turn causes more avoidance, and couples get stuck in this cycle. This pattern of what couples themselves might view as infrequent sex is common, with roughly one in five couples being sexual fewer than 10 times per year.

How have you and your partner handled occasions when one of you wanted to engage sexually but the other preferred not to at that time? Did you feel good about who initiated on different occasions? Have there been times when you and your partner went without being sexually intimate for much longer than either of you wanted? Has the frequency of your sexual interactions in the past six months changed significantly from earlier in your relationship? If so, did either of you express concern about this, and how did the other respond?

Dissatisfaction with the Quality of Sexual Intimacy. You and your partner may vary in what you find to be sexually appealing. For some people, the quality of sex depends heavily on the level of romance—for example, soft music, candles, or nonsexual intimacy beforehand. For others, sexual intimacy is heightened by the experience of mutual physical passion during sexual activity. Some people enjoy sex most when they've been able to anticipate it throughout the day, using touches or glances as reminders of the intent to be sexual later that evening; others enjoy sex most when it's unplanned and spontaneous. Partners don't always agree on what they find sexually exciting or even comfortable, and these differences can be difficult to navigate.

Couples sometimes struggle under the pressure to achieve "great sex" every time they're sexually intimate. Although experiences vary widely among couples, for many couples about 40–50% of sexual experiences are very good for both partners; 20–25% are very good for one partner and fine for the other. About 20–25% of sexual exchanges are reported as acceptable but not remarkable, and the remaining 10–15% are mediocre or unsatisfying. Thus, a range in quality of sexual experiences is completely normal. Failure to recognize this variety in sexual experiences within the same relationship can lead either partner to feel unnecessary disappointment, frustration, guilt, or resentment. Prior to the affair, did either or both of you experience dissatisfaction with the quality of your sexual interactions?

Difficulties in Talking About Sex. You and your partner might experience difficulties in talking about your sexual relationship. This isn't unusual, because many people come to believe that sex should simply happen naturally and couples shouldn't need to talk about it. For example, you might have difficulty in expressing your feelings about sex, or your partner may have difficulty in listening or responding to these feelings in a supportive way. Some couples are able to communicate effectively about anything *except* sex. Or discussions about sexual difficulties may occur primarily in bed, when one partner is feeling particularly frustrated, and these conversations may not be constructive.

Have you and your partner had difficulties talking about aspects of your own sexual relationship—for example, about how often to make love or about your respective likes and dislikes? When you experienced differences, did you go about finding compromises and, if so, how? How would you need to change your own role to initiate or take part in discussions about your sexual relationship for these to go better?

Barriers to Sexual Intimacy. Even if you and your partner both have similar sexual drives and preferences, other factors can serve as barriers to sexual intimacy. For example, one of the most common barriers that couples describe involves time pressures resulting from work and raising children. Another common barrier to sexual intimacy involves issues of physical and emotional health. Some people don't enjoy having sex if they're struggling with allergies, chronic pain, or physical fatigue. Others are almost always ready to engage in sex, even if they've had a bad day. Sexual desire, arousal, and performance are often affected by emotional factors such as anxiety or depression—as well as by medications commonly used to treat these conditions.

Perhaps you or your partner struggles with specific sexual difficulties. If so, you're not alone. Common problems for partners include difficulties becoming aroused or maintaining physical arousal even if you have sexual desire, difficulties around having an orgasm—either too quickly or not at all—or pain during intercourse. A large proportion of people, perhaps up to half, may experience one of these specific sexual problems at some time or another. Interestingly, specific sexual problems are often unrelated to sexual satisfaction or overall happiness in the relationship. It's only when these problems contribute to additional feelings such as not being desired or cared for that couples experience higher risk for becoming emotionally and physically disconnected.

What role do you and your partner want sexual intimacy to have in your relationship, and are there barriers to sexual intimacy that you and your partner have experienced? Knowing what you know now, how could you reduce these obstacles to sexual intimacy as a couple? Exercise 6.4 is designed to help you consider how difficulties in physical connection may have made your relationship more vulnerable to an affair, as well as ways of promoting physical intimacy in moving forward if that's a goal that you have.

Were We Ever a Healthy Couple?

In the initial chaos following an affair, it's easy to lose a broader view of your relationship from a long-term perspective. As an injured partner, it may be difficult to recall earlier times when you were confident in the love and commitment you experienced because right now you feel deeply hurt. Or you may now view those earlier feelings with suspicion, perhaps doubting your judgment or questioning how truthful your partner has ever been with you. As an involved partner, it may be difficult to focus on what you've valued most in your relationship because it seems at such odds with your decision to have an affair.

In evaluating whether you can make this relationship work again—and whether you even want to—you need not only to consider what was happening in the few months leading up to the affair but also to ask some questions about the broader picture of your relationship from its beginning (listed in the box on the facing page and discussed below). What were the good reasons for becoming a couple? What have been your most worthwhile times together? There may also have been some important vulnerabilities in your relationship from the outset or others that have been around for some time. You need to examine the foundation of this relationship from early on to examine what vulnerabilities may be long-term, how to address them, and how difficult those vulnerabilities might be to change.

Questions to consider when viewing your relationship from the broader perspective include the following:

- Why did we become a couple?
- How satisfied were we with our respective roles?
- What have we done well?
- What challenges have we overcome in the past?
- How does the current crisis fit into the big picture?
- What would it take to restore or create a strong relationship now?

Why Did We Become a Couple?

What attracted you and your partner to each other? Couples often describe finding the other person easy to talk to and physically attractive, sharing fun times together, or having a good sexual relationship. Other common reasons include having similar interests or backgrounds or sharing important values. What led to your decision to commit to one another? Do you value the same parts of the relationship now as you did then?

Relationships mature and need to accommodate change, just as people do. You may have entered your relationship based on qualities that worked well then but don't serve it as well now. Or perhaps there were initial sources of attraction or reasons for becoming a couple that weren't entirely healthy. For example, was either of you drawn to the other primarily from a fear of growing older without a partner or children? Or did you enter this relationship in part to escape a difficult family situation? You may recognize now that there were early warning signs in your relationship that you either missed or ignored. For example, maybe your courtship was chaotic, with repeated breakups or threats to end the relationship. The fact that your relationship may not have been great from the beginning doesn't mean you can't improve it now. It can simply be important to evaluate whether you've had a good relationship in the past and somehow got off track or you need to build a strong foundation now for the first time.

No partner is perfect. Successful relationships are those in which partners grow together despite their shortcomings, care for each other despite their flaws and differences, and nurture their respective strengths to hold on to the positive and minimize the negative. What were the good qualities that drew you to each other? Were there fundamental flaws in your relationship or in each other that you overlooked? What would it take to recover the best parts of your relationship and each other that, at one time, made you want to spend the rest of your lives together?

How Satisfied Were We with Our Respective Roles?

You or your partner may have committed to your relationship with one set of expectations, only to discover later that your experience ended up quite different. The arrival of children, financial setbacks, or unexpected challenges related to physical health or other concerns can all dramatically change partners' roles in and outside their home. Even the best-laid-out plans can be disrupted by circumstances that neither one of you could have anticipated. Or perhaps you or your partner never discussed your expectations about your respective roles in your relationship. Even if you both felt quite pleased with your roles at some point in your relationship, as you go through life, you and your partner might change and no longer find those same roles rewarding, or find that new roles don't fit well for one or both of you.

Disappointments from unmet expectations can easily lead to discontent or resentment more broadly. Consider the roles you and your partner have most recently had in your relationship as a wage earner, house or family manager, intimate partner, parent, or caretaker for another person. Has either of you felt frustrated or believed you had less opportunity than the other in areas that were important to you? Were you able to talk about these challenges in ways that felt mutually understanding and supportive? If you're particularly unhappy with the roles you've had, what would you need to do to change these roles and what assistance would you need from your partner?

What Have We Done Well?

What stand out as the best parts of your relationship? Despite the trauma of an affair and earlier struggles, couples can often identify aspects of their experience that stand out as particularly worthwhile or special—for example, raising their children together or working as a team to build a business or create a comfortable home. For some, the best parts of being a couple have been about friendship or mutual support during times of crisis. What would you have missed out on if you hadn't become a couple? What would you miss if you ended your relationship now?

As you reflect on the best parts of your relationship in the past, how did these come about? For example, did they happen spontaneously by being yourselves? Or did some of your prior success as a couple require conscious effort and determination? It will probably require hard work to put your relationship back on solid ground again, if that's the course you decide to pursue. There may be times when you feel as though you're losing ground rather than gaining. However, it may be easier to maintain efforts to rebuild this relationship if you can recall some of your best times in the past as well as how you managed to achieve them. You'll also need to decide how much you want to "go back to how we were in the past" versus using this recovery process as a possible opportunity to change your relationship in new, constructive ways.

What Challenges Have We Overcome?

Prior to the affair, you and your partner may already have gone through times that were difficult or challenging. For example, you may have faced financial crises, high demands from rearing children, dealing with illness experienced by one of you or a family member, loss of a job, or a move to a different part of the country. Such challenges can strain a relationship in ways that weaken it or leave lasting disappointments or resentments. However, often couples can look back on such occasions with some satisfaction in recognizing that they withstood the challenge and perhaps even emerged stronger.

What have been the most difficult times you and your partner have faced together before this affair? What strategies did you draw on to make it through your most challenging times? Can you recall times in the past when either one of you felt deeply hurt or disappointed by the other? If so, how did you deal with those occasions? You may never have experienced a hurt in your relationship that comes close to the pain you're feeling now. Nevertheless, thinking about times when you've been able to work through hurt feelings together and to move forward—even for lesser relationship injuries—may offer insight into strategies you could draw on as a couple for working through this crisis.

How Does the Current Crisis Fit into the Big Picture?

People *are* capable of change. The important questions to consider are what changes are needed, whether you are both committed to those changes, and how realistic it is to make these specific changes. When injured partners struggle to determine whether they could ever feel secure again, we encourage them to look at the big picture of their relationship. Has your partner been faithful and truthful in the past prior to this affair? Has your partner been able to take responsibility for hurtful actions in the past and successfully commit to changing? If relationship problems left your relationship more vulnerable to an affair, are these problems fairly recent or have they been there from the beginning?

If you're the person who had the affair, you also need to view your relationship and your partner within the bigger picture. The emotional turmoil and conflict that follow an affair may not provide an accurate picture of what your relationship was like before the affair or what it could be like down the road if you and your partner decide to stay together and work through this challenge. It's not fair to your partner and not in your own best interests to make a decision about what to do with your relationship based on what's going on now. A better basis for evaluating the future requires looking at the big picture, including a recognition of times that felt the best as well as times when you struggled together through the worst.

What Would It Take to Build a Strong Relationship Now?

Abby and Colin, the couple described earlier in this chapter, spent many long hours exploring how their relationship had become vulnerable. Abby recognized that by allowing herself to become totally absorbed in her role at home as the family manager, she had cut herself off from important sources of emotional support from close friends she had known for years. She learned to approach Colin in a softer tone when conveying her needs for closeness and to provide *him with encouragement when he felt overwhelmed at work or ineffective at home. Colin worked hard at being more receptive to suggestions from Abby about how to handle the boys when they were upset or difficult to manage. He also learned to listen more supportively to Abby's feelings of frustration without becoming defensive or feeling he was necessarily to blame.*

Over time, Colin and Abby began to rebuild their relationship. They made relationship time a priority. Together they reached decisions regarding finances and child care that allowed Abby to resume a role in their business one afternoon each week while Colin took the boys on a prearranged outing. During the first six months, they both continued to wrestle with difficult feelings of hurt, guilt, and apprehension about their future together. Their relationship went through numerous ups and downs. But their commitment and efforts at identifying vulnerabilities in their relationship and making critical changes eventually paid off. A year after Abby's affair, they had worked through the crisis and had found ways to change their roles at home and grow closer as a couple.

As you've examined your relationship in more detail, what vulnerabilities have you identified? What relationship strengths have you also recognized—either now or in the past? Unless you've already decided to end your relationship, identify everything you can do on your own to reduce unnecessary conflict and to create an environment that enables both you and your partner to achieve greater fulfillment in your roles in and outside the home. Then commit yourself to implementing as many changes as you can on your own for a specific time period (for example, 30 or 90 days). During this time, look for opportunities to work on the relationship together with your partner and use every chance you find to work together. When the opportunities aren't there, try to work on behalf of the relationship on your own. A useful way of expressing your intentions to your partner may be something like this:

"I know that this is a really difficult time for us. I still want us to see whether we can find ways of making our relationship work. For now, I'm going to work hard at being a better partner. Sometimes I'll probably fall short, but I'm going to continue trying anyway. I'm also hoping that a part of you still wants our relationship to work too, and that there will be

ways that we can work together. I'll try to be clearer about what I need from you, and I hope you'll be open about what you need from me."

As you work on strengthening your relationship, look for evidence that your efforts are having an impact. For example, do you feel better about yourself, have greater confidence in your ability to influence what's happening in your life, or respect yourself more? Do your efforts appear to be having an impact on your partner? Have you acknowledged your partner's efforts as a way of encouraging them further? Are your conflicts any less frequent or less intense? Are there any ways in which you and your partner seem closer or have been more able to work together as a team?

Anticipate that any progress you make in your relationship will be accompanied by occasional setbacks. It's often impossible to know what you're capable of as a couple until you both make strong efforts to change. Making that effort is an important part of showing both of you what your potential as a couple might be. If you can hang in there and get through these struggles, you and your partner may be able to make some important and lasting positive steps toward building a stronger relationship together. If not, that will become more evident. In any case, making the effort first puts you in a better position to make important decisions about the future of your relationship.

EXERCISES

EXERCISE 6.1 Identifying What You Hope to Gain from This Process

Decide what you hope to gain from exploring the affair and trying to understand why it happened. For example, as the injured partner you might be thinking:

> *"I need to understand why this happened because I can't make any sense of our relationship right now. If I understand better why it happened, then maybe I can evaluate whether it's likely to happen again or how we need to change things."*

Or as the involved partner you might think:

"I never thought I'd do this. I need to get a better understanding of how this happened to know whether my partner and I can make the changes we need to make for our relationship to work."

Write down at least two things you hope to gain by exploring why the affair occurred. Then share these objectives with your partner and discuss why you need to understand what happened and how you believe it will benefit each of you.

EXERCISE 6.2 Identifying and Dealing with Conflict

Identify major sources of conflict in your relationship, whether these are certain aspects of either one of you, how you interact as a couple, or how you interact with people outside your relationship that contribute to this conflict. Clarify which of these conflicts were present prior to the affair and which ones have emerged since then. For example, perhaps you've always struggled with conflict over how to save or spend money, or now tensions arise when one of your friends offers unsolicited advice on how to deal with issues between the two of you. Knowing how long the problem has existed might give you some sense of how difficult it will be to change.

Recognizing what creates conflict between the two of you is important, but doing something about it is critical if you want to stay in your relationship and make it as good as possible. For each of the sources of conflict you identified earlier, describe what you can do, either individually or as a couple, to address the conflict more effectively. For example, if a major conflict involves how your respective friends get too involved in your issues as a couple, you might decide that each of you will have an individual talk with your friends to let them know what kinds of support you find helpful, but that you and your partner have to figure out how to deal with your couple issues on your own.

EXERCISE 6.3 Promoting Emotional Intimacy

List the major ways that you and your partner have interacted in the past that led to feeling emotionally close. Some of these may have been disrupted by the affair, but think back to your relationship before that time. For example:

"I often felt closest when we just got silly with each other around the house. Sometimes when music was playing in the background, we'd break into dance and then go back to our chores. I could never do that with anyone else."

There might also be ways of feeling close that you haven't experienced in the past or that you'd like to develop further. List ways you'd like to explore to create more emotional closeness and specific plans for developing these. For example:

"We used to talk about our dreams and what we wanted for a life together. Now it seems we just try to get through each day. I'd like us to create a new future together by sitting down at least once a month and 'dreaming' together over a cup of coffee with no one else around."

EXERCISE 6.4 Promoting Physical Intimacy

List the major ways that you and your partner have been physically affectionate in the past that led to feelings of closeness. For example:

"One of my favorite times has been in the mornings when we would wake up and snuggle for a few minutes. I need that to start the day and feel connected when we're apart."

Suggest some additional ways of showing affection. For example:

"I'd really like it if we would hold hands when we're walking someplace. And when we're home and watching TV, I'd like to sit close together on the sofa or lie in bed together and watch our favorite shows."

Also describe what you've enjoyed about your sexual relationship in the past or ways you'd like to improve it. For example:

"More and more, it seems that either one of us is too tired or distracted to engage in sex. At least once in a while I'd like to try planning for sexual intimacy ahead of time, so we can set aside a better time and not be tired or distracted."

7

Was It the World around Us?

Like many couples, Ira and Hannah struggled to keep up with their busy lives. Full-time jobs and three children left no room for a social life and barely allowed time for dinner or a movie every few weeks. Ira had taken on extra responsibilities at work and rarely made it home for dinner. Hannah spent evenings monitoring the kids' homework and catching up on chores after a full day of teaching. After 19 years of marriage, they felt like the proverbial ships that pass in the night, and their sex life had all but evaporated. They talked about their drifting apart and resolved to change things but usually felt too tired or stressed to follow through.

Ira sometimes found it easier to talk to his office mate at work, Morgan, whose husband was often away on business trips. Over time, they began to talk about their marriages and their frustrations, although they were clear with each other about being committed to their partners. Their affair seemed to sneak up on them after weeks of laughing at each other's jokes, sitting a bit too close, and then touching hands a bit longer than necessary when Morgan passed materials to Ira in their office. When their relationship eventually became sexual, both expressed guilt; at different times both tried to pull back from the affair, but each time they felt drawn back in.

Hannah sensed a growing distance from Ira. When he started coming home later and later, she confronted him, and Ira acknowledged the affair but insisted he would break it off if Hannah could just forgive him. Neither Ira nor Hannah wanted their marriage to end. They just weren't sure they could ever make it right again.

When people enter a committed relationship and pledge to remain faithful, they usually mean it. But relationships become vulnerable. They can become weakened from the outside just as they can be weakened from within. During the first few years of a typical relationship, life together can be relatively simple. There may be few financial stressors; an absence of children may leave you plenty of time for each other, and possibly your jobs and careers haven't overloaded you with responsibilities yet. You might be young and healthy at that point; you may have few outside commitments to your community, and your parents may not have reached a stage of their lives where they're beginning to depend on you.

Enter time and the complications of life. If you have children now, you know how much time and energy they need and deserve. We don't have to list the expenses that you've added to your budget or the obligations you've added to your daily schedule. Life has become fuller but also possibly harder. In and of themselves, these normal, predictable challenges rarely cause committed couple relationships to fail. However, when several stressors occur in combination, they can take a heavy toll on the amount and quality of time that partners have for their own relationship. As you consider the common outside influences described below (and listed in the box below), and as you work through Exercise 7.1, ask yourself the following:

Did time and energy devoted elsewhere place our relationship at risk?

Common outside intrusions into a couple's relationship include the following:

- Work-related demands on time and energy

- Responsibilities of raising children

- Outside commitments such as volunteer work or activism

- Responsibilities to extended family or friends—including frequent gatherings or caring for ill or aging family members

- Household tasks

- Hobbies and interests

How can we minimize these intrusions to safeguard and nurture our relationship?

How Did Outside Intrusions Come between Us?

Work

People vary in how much their work defines how they feel about themselves. When work forms a large part of your identity or how you see yourself, it's easy for that part of life to dominate other parts. Even if you're working from home or part-time, you may spend increasingly long hours focused on work-related responsibilities and wind up being distracted or emotionally unavailable to your partner.

Work can be seductive. Sometimes we understand better how to do our work than how to be the kind of partner our relationship needs or the caregiver our children need. And the rewards from work are sometimes more immediate and more tangible. We're encouraged to work hard and get ahead, but this can easily become a vicious cycle. The harder we work and the more successful we are, the greater the incentives to work harder to achieve even more—whether this means achieving financial rewards, recognition from others, or simply a sense of personal accomplishment.

In our role as couple therapists, our clients often tell us they work so hard because they have to. They have to support the family. If they let up at work, they and their families will suffer. Bills won't get paid, or there won't be family vacations, or college for their children will be out of the question. In most cases, there's just enough truth in each of these assertions to create a sense of being trapped. After all, bills *do* have to get paid. But in every case, there's also a choice being made. If by working so hard to support your family you end up *losing* your family because your relationship becomes more vulnerable to an affair, is the effort worth it?

What would you be willing to give up in terms of your work for the sake of your relationship? What limits are you willing to set on the time and energy you devote to work to redirect your focus to nurturing your relationship? What specific steps would you have to take to implement these limits? How can you increase support at work or at home for your decision to place your relationship as a highest priority?

Responsibilities of Raising Children

Next to work, raising children is the most frequently cited demand on couples' time. And each stage of child rearing can compete with a couple's relationship time in different ways. Raising children can be so demanding and so exhausting that the *only* way to do this well is to make sure that as a couple you preserve time and energy for your own relationship. *One of the best gifts that parents can give to their children is a secure home in which the parents love and nurture one another as an example of a loving relationship for their children.* Placing your own relationship at risk by devoting all your time and energy to your children at the expense of partners' caring for each other just doesn't work. Parents need to risk their children's frustrations or disappointments in the short run by setting aside time for themselves as a couple to promote their children's well-being in the long run. Not only is it developmentally healthy for kids to experience some frustration and to learn that their needs are not the center of the parental universe, but your modeling how to care for yourselves and your relationship is important for your child's long-term growth and future relationships.

Balancing your commitments to your children and to your relationship requires continuous effort. For example, it might include partnering with other couples to trade evenings of providing child care. Or it may involve helping your children understand that their parents need separate time together before joining in family time. Above all, it requires a steady commitment to setting aside quality time for you and your partner and placing your own relationship as a top priority—not because you don't care about your children, but specifically because you *do* care for them. By giving your relationship a high priority, you're showing how to have a healthy and loving adult intimate relationship. Modeling this is as important as being physically engaged with your children. They won't be harmed if you take time for your partner; more likely, they'll benefit.

In what ways have the demands of child rearing disrupted time and energy you and your partner set aside for yourselves as a couple? For example, if you've allowed your children to participate in so many activities outside of school that these consume your available time as well as theirs, how can you scale back? Identify resources you could draw on to provide respite and opportunities to focus on your relationship as a couple. What steps could you take to ensure that you and your partner have at least a brief amount of quiet time together each day to talk by yourselves and reconnect with each other?

Outside Commitments

It's not just work or children that compete for your time and energy. Numerous groups, such as your children's schools, religious organizations, political activities, or various community service organizations, depend on the contributions of volunteers. At appropriate levels, the satisfaction derived from contributing to such causes can not only enrich individual lives but also bring outside energy into the home. As with work, however, it's a matter of balance and priorities.

How much time do you and your partner devote to commitments outside the home other than work? In what ways have such commitments interfered with time for your own relationship? What limits would you need to set on outside commitments to reduce the risks posed to your relationship by spending too much time apart?

Responsibilities to Extended Family or Friends

For many couples, partners' respective families of origin or close long-term friendships provide an important source of emotional and other support. At the same time, involvement with extended family or close friends can create additional demands or strains. It's not uncommon for partners to have different expectations about how much time or energy to devote to their own or to each other's extended family and vital friendships. Such differences can lead to resentment about feeling like less of a priority in your partner's life or about feeling denied the opportunity to hold on to important emotional ties with others.

Another way in which responsibilities to others can strain a couple's relationship occurs when one or the other partner takes on a caregiving role for someone in the extended family. A common example involves caring for an aging parent, but it can just as easily involve caring for grandparents or siblings with physical or mental challenges. Partners engaged in such caregiving often have a profound sense of responsibility deeply rooted in admirable family values. However, as in caring for one's children, it's important to maintain a balance that also protects and nurtures the couple's own relationship.

In what ways have your or your partner's involvement with extended family or close friends detracted from the time and energy you've devoted to your own relationship? If your involvement comes from caregiving responsibilities, how can you redesign your roles to set reasonable limits that will preserve vital emotional and time resources for your own relationship? What additional resources could you draw on to balance these commitments and relationships more effectively?

Household Tasks

All couples have ongoing responsibilities in the home as well. Obvious tasks include laundry, cleaning, meals, house or car maintenance, yard work, paying the bills, and so forth. Even when you and your partner agree on how to divide or share these responsibilities, getting everything done while preserving time for your relationship can seem impossible. When you disagree on how to share these tasks or one of you feels the other isn't upholding their end of the bargain, resentment often follows. Moreover, you and your partner might agree on how to divide household tasks but disagree on how to get them done or how important they are compared with reserving time simply to relax or play together.

In thinking about how you and your partner manage household tasks, consider these questions: Do you generally agree on how to divide up household tasks, or does either of you frequently feel you do more than your share? How willing are you to put work at home aside to preserve time to relax and play together? How could you and your partner collaborate to balance work and play at home in ways that feel better for both of you? Do household tasks leave either of you so exhausted that you have little energy left for your relationship?

Hobbies and Interests

Hobbies and leisure activities can reduce stress and increase emotional and physical well-being, make a person more interesting to be around, and even promote shared recreation when the two of you are interested in the same thing. But they can become a distraction when they take up too much time, especially when you already have too little time for each other.

> Alondra loved the energy and health benefits she gained by working out, so she devoted an hour each day after work to it and at least half a day each weekend. Devon resented the time he spent alone at home but didn't want to join Alondra at the gym. He had always had an interest in rebuilding cars, and before long he and his friends were traveling on weekends to auto shows out of town. Neither Devon nor Alondra wanted to give up their own outside interests, even when it became clear they were spending too little time together for several weeks in a row.

In what ways have you or your partner allowed hobbies or similar interests to come between you, and how could you change that? How willing are you to scale back the amount of time you devote to separate interests? Could either of you become more accepting of separate hobbies if you were also spending more time together?

How Did Stress Overcome Us?

Low levels of stress or more serious but temporary stressors are often manageable and can even be positive if they cause you to think or behave in new ways that are better for you in the long run. But when stress is severe or long-term, it can cause bigger and longer-lasting problems, including in your relationship.

Excessive or prolonged stress can place a relationship at higher risk for an affair when the stressors cause partners to neglect themselves or their relationship. Common sources of stress that can damage your relationship are listed in the box on the next page. Sometimes a partner under duress tries to escape emotionally into the comfort of an affair relationship that is largely sheltered from day-to-day realities. Other times a partner overwhelmed by stress becomes emotionally or physically unavailable, leaving the other partner feeling abandoned and vulnerable to the attention of someone else. When stress permeates a household, both partners can become irritable and impatient, more likely to fault each other for

Common sources of stress that can undermine a relationship include the following:

- Chronic financial strains
- Demanding life transitions—for example, becoming parents or starting a new job
- Chronic health problems
- Ongoing conflicts with others—for example, with extended family or coworkers
- Experiences of marginalization, prejudice, or discrimination as individuals or as a couple
- Strains within the broader community including crime, social or political unrest, pandemics, or natural disasters

problems neither is really responsible for, and gradually they decline into a cycle of mutual blame and resentment.

Stress from Marginalization or Discrimination

Some couples encounter significant stress from experiences of marginalization or discrimination within their community. For example, individuals who are members of ethnic, sexual, gender, or religious minorities might experience various forms of discrimination ranging from smaller daily slights to more explicit forms of discrimination. Other couples may experience discrimination or marginalization based on certain aspects of their identities. For example, if the two partners have different skin tones, others might respond to them negatively. Or if the two partners differ noticeably in age, either strangers or family may be unsupportive of the relationship, assuming that one or both partners must have some "unresolved issues." In some communities, committing to a partner of a different religious faith may lead to exclusion from various family or social events or prompt suggestions that one partner would be better off with someone "more appropriate." These and similar stressors from the broader community can challenge partners, erode their emotional resources, deprive them of important social support, and—eventually—render them less resilient to other factors that increase vulnerability to an affair.

Over the past year, how has stress made your relationship vulnerable? Which stressors developed gradually or escaped your notice until it seemed too late? What would be required now to reduce or eliminate the sources of greatest stress? What additional resources can you draw on for help?

> Ira and Hannah, the couple described at the beginning of this chapter, took a hard look at how they had allowed outside demands to erode their emotional connection. In trying so hard to be responsible providers for their family, they had neglected to care for their own relationship. Both began to impose more effective limits on their work. They also reassigned responsibilities in the home to each of the children—including having their teenage son babysit for his younger siblings one night each week so the couple could go out by themselves. Ira and Hannah identified certain days during the week that were particularly stressful for one of them or the other and agreed to exchange "care days" on those occasions so each could get some relief when it was needed most. They also pursued more intentional touching and hugging throughout the day. Their increased commitment to nurturing their relationship didn't by itself solve the deep hurt caused by Ira's affair, but it gave both partners increased hope that they could collaborate in creating a stronger relationship and moving forward together.

Did We Let Others Undermine Our Relationship?

Vows exchanged by partners when they formalize a committed relationship typically include promises of fidelity—"forsaking all others." It's ironic, then, how frequently sexual infidelity is portrayed in our culture through books, movies, and other media as commonplace, romantic, and often without severe negative effects. At times infidelity almost seems taken for granted—depicted in a glamorous or even comical way—rather than being portrayed in a more realistic manner as a relationship trauma with devastating personal and relationship consequences. Anyone's commitment to fidelity can be undermined when we are continually exposed to this perspective.

Most of Mateo's friends at work were still single. On Fridays after work, they all had a ritual of going out together to a local bar. Often the other guys would flirt with women and would tease Mateo about being "tied down" and missing out on life. Mateo had always felt thankful for his and Brianna's relationship, and he couldn't imagine a life without her. But things started to change after their first child arrived. Brianna resented the time Mateo spent with his friends because she was often at home taking care of the baby after work and hadn't seen her friends in weeks. When they were home together, Brianna was short-tempered with Mateo and didn't seem to want to spend time with him, which confused Mateo. His friends at work teased him even more when he talked about the problems at home. One of his friends and two women from work invited him out for drinks one evening, and eventually they started going out once a week.

One evening Mateo and Nicole, who had recently divorced, went out after work for drinks by themselves when their friends weren't available. Mateo didn't intend for anything to happen between him and Nicole—he just enjoyed talking with her. Eventually he and Nicole were going out after work every few weeks by themselves. When Nicole invited Mateo over to her apartment instead of going to the bar, he felt flattered. When they got to her apartment and she kissed him, he was a bit surprised and initially resisted going further. But Nicole continued to hold him and caress his neck, and eventually led him to her bedroom. That was the first of several such episodes that continued for several months.

People like Mateo, with no prior intention of becoming involved in an affair, often become more vulnerable to participating in one after repeated exposure to flirtation or outright pursuit by an outsider. Only with 20/20 hindsight do they recognize, once they've had an affair, all the temptations and fidelity-undermining messages they've been barraged with. It's worth examining the common sources of temptation and other negative influences discussed below to see which contributed to the affair that disrupted your relationship so that you or your partner won't be so vulnerable to these forces again. As the injured partner, you'll benefit from understanding potential risk factors that contributed to your partner's affair and should read this section. But most of this next section is aimed at encouraging involved partners to explore how they may not have maintained boundaries that would prevent outside influences from undermining their commitment to fidelity. When we say "you" here, we're speaking to *involved* partners.

General Temptations and Opportunity

In working with involved partners, we sometimes ask, "How did you reach your decision to have an affair?" A common response is "I never decided to have an affair—it just happened." Our next question—admittedly more difficult to answer—is "Well, how is it you failed to reach a decision *not* to have an affair?" The implication is that you can identify risky situations ahead of time and take explicit steps to avoid these. Consider the following situations that present either temptation or opportunity for an affair:

- Mason's work in sales frequently requires him to travel to cities in which he has no friends, family, or colleagues. After working long days, he usually has dinner at a local bar or dance club.

- Paige has been spending lots of time over the past few months preparing for a school carnival with Nate, a single parent from her daughter's school whose work schedule allows him to spend much of his day at home.

- Tuan and Lily have been working nights and weekends on a remodeling project for a local business. No one else is involved in the project, and sometimes they take time out at the restaurant down the street before returning to work—without informing their partners later.

Do any of these situations have elements that seem familiar? We're not suggesting that any of these scenarios is inherently wrong, but we *are* saying that people need to recognize the possible temptations in a situation—no matter how far-fetched they may seem ahead of time—and then set clear boundaries to ensure that temptations or risky situations don't lead to poor decisions. Some questions to help you determine whether an outside relationship could lead to risks or temptation are listed in the box on the next page.

Related questions to consider are whether you've taken steps to protect your relationship from such risks. For example, if you're traveling alone,

If you're uncertain whether an outside relationship has begun to edge toward a "special" friendship that poses a risk, ask yourself the following:

- Would you be willing to change the nature of this outside friendship (for example, give it up or limit it) for the sake of your own committed relationship? If not, there's a good chance that it has already developed a "romantic specialness" that may threaten emotional or physical bonds your partner regards as unique to your own relationship.

- Would you be willing to talk with the other person about the "mixed signals" you're getting about the boundaries of your friendship— knowing that they might then pull back from the relationship you're currently enjoying? Are there elements of flirtation or emotional closeness that have already become something you look forward to and would miss if they ended?

- Are there *any* aspects of your interactions with the outside person you'd be reluctant for your partner to know about or that you're *hiding* or *deliberately not telling* your partner? Are there any discussions you would not disclose fully to your partner? Would you be uncomfortable receiving a phone call or text from the outside person when you're with your partner?

do you make it a point to call your partner regularly to stay emotionally connected and to keep your relationship at the forefront of your thoughts? Do you make sure that people you meet know that you're married or in a committed relationship? If your partner is frequently out of town, do you draw on friends in committed relationships to keep you company or to socialize? If your work or involvement in the community results in your spending time with a coworker, have you taken steps to ensure that feelings of personal closeness don't develop to an inappropriate level or cascade into feelings of strong sexual attraction? For example, do you limit highly personal discussions or other intimate exchanges with your coworker that could lead to an inappropriate level of intimacy?

Take a hard, close look at how you and your partner spend your time whenever you're apart. What opportunities might either of you face that could increase the risk of infidelity? Some risky situations are obvious, but others might depend on you and your own vulnerabilities. An important part of identifying and dealing with risky situations is *knowing yourself.* What is it that you find attractive in people *in general*? How have you built closeness with others in the past? What situations might be particularly risky for you? For example, if you've always been drawn to people with a sense of humor, you need to remain mindful if you and an attractive new coworker discover that you have the same sense of humor through daily office banter. Identifying such situations doesn't indicate your interest in an affair; rather, identifying potentially risky situations and taking active measures to keep these situations safe conveys your commitment *not* to have an affair and to remove opportunities or temptations to behave in ways that jeopardize your relationship.

Pursuit by an Outsider

It feels good to feel attractive or desirable. We all like to receive compliments. "Innocent" flirtation often feels good for similar reasons. It can be reassuring to know that someone else considers us charming, emotionally sensitive, physically attractive, or whatever other characteristic we'd like to believe we have. It feels especially good to receive such compliments when we tend toward self-doubt or haven't been receiving such comments from our partner.

It's not unusual to be drawn into an affair following pursuit by someone outside the relationship. Such pursuit may develop gradually over months or even years of interaction, or it may come quite unexpectedly from an acquaintance. The pursuit may begin with an explicit intention by the other to have an affair or as a genuine wish to have a special friendship based on caring and trust that subsequently leads to feelings of strong physical or emotional attraction. Sometimes an outsider persists despite clear, explicit resistance and discouragement. And other times a pursuit continues because of an individual's tolerance or subtle encouragement.

To reduce vulnerability to outsiders who may wish to pursue an affair—or who may simply be "receptive" to such a relationship—it's important to remain vigilant. That doesn't mean rejecting all friendships with colleagues, friends, and others. It doesn't mean rejecting all expressions of caring or interpreting them as implicit sexual advances. But it does mean being clear about the boundaries of such relationships—that you don't pursue or accept suggestions of separate time together in inappropriate settings, that you guard against personal discussions that push a friendship to a deeper emotional level that goes beyond appropriate boundaries, and that you commit to never keeping interactions with others secret from your partner.

We've counseled people who insisted on retaining a risky outside relationship because it was an "innocent friendship and was not sexual." In most cases, their reluctance to relinquish the outside friendship indicated that the other person had already become emotionally important to them. Emotional closeness to others isn't a problem on its own. However, if your partner raises concerns about a particular outside relationship, there's a possibility that something about that relationship poses a potential risk, and the two of you could benefit from discussing it further. Being emotionally close to someone else doesn't mean you've decided to have an affair. It's simply that an affair *sometimes* develops when a person views an outside relationship as "safe" and then gradually becomes more emotionally involved with the other person without maintaining necessary limits or boundaries. One test of whether your outside relationship is risky is to ask yourself if you're keeping **any** aspect of it hidden from your partner. If you are, then it's likely that you've already crossed an emotional boundary, even if that relationship hasn't yet become physical.

Where you decide to set limits on how you and your partner interact with others depends on what the two of you choose to keep exclusive between you. In consensual monogamous relationships, having sexual interactions or falling in love with someone else is unacceptable. However, some couples may remain committed to each other but agree to "open up" certain aspects of their relationship including intimate interactions with others. This might include sexual behaviors with or romantic feelings for other people—what's sometimes referred to as an open, nonmonogamous, or polyamorous relationship. What's important is that *you and your partner agree on shared boundaries* and are able to live within those boundaries in a healthy manner. Regardless of where a couple sets specific boundaries around their relationship, those boundaries can still be crossed and infidelity can occur in any kind of relationship. An example of infidelity in a nonmonogamous relationship might involve complications when one partner's relationship with an outside person gradually evolves beyond what the couple agreed to on either an emotional or a physical level. It's important for couples who are engaged in relationships that include others in various intimate ways to be clear about the boundaries of those relationships, high-risk situations, and the evolving desires and goals of the other persons outside of the previously agreed-upon boundaries.

Friends and Acquaintances Who Devalue Fidelity

No one has a greater investment in preserving your relationship than you and your partner do. Unfortunately, not only may your friends or acquaintances fail to actively promote your remaining faithful, they may either actively or indirectly discourage it. Like Mateo's friends described earlier, they may encourage you to party with them and tease you if you state that you "need to call home" first. They may encourage you to go to singles bars because "a little looking never hurt anyone." Or they may serve as a "go-between" for someone outside your relationship who has expressed an interest in you or try to "set you up" with someone else they think is better for you.

Other means of undermining your fidelity are less direct. For example, your single or divorced friends may talk up all the benefits of being single while ignoring the downsides. They may listen to your own stories of unhappiness in your relationship and encourage your feelings of unfairness by siding with you in an unbalanced way. Or they may undermine your relationship by competing for time you would otherwise spend with your partner.

How Should We Draw on Others to Support Our Relationship?

It's not enough to protect yourself from outside influences that undermine your relationship. You also can benefit from seeking out support from sources that actively nurture your relationship and *reduce* its vulnerability. What bases of support for fidelity and for your relationship in general are available to you and your partner? Although such assets vary in couples' lives, some common resources are described here. Exercise 7.2 will help you consider specific resources in your own life.

Couple Friends

Developing friendships with other committed couples can provide an important source of caring and support for your own relationship. What couples do you know who enjoy spending time with each other—partners who are courteous to one another, laugh with each other, express their complaints respectfully, tolerate each other's shortcomings, and work together at overcoming occasional disappointments or irritations? Your own relationship can be strengthened by spending time with couples whose values are similar to those you aspire to yourself. Avoid couples who constantly bicker, put each other down, are generally insensitive to one another, or appear to pursue individual interests that put their relationship at risk; hanging out with these kinds of couples can increase the likelihood of you seeing these kinds of interactions as acceptable and normal, which in turn can create more risk for your own relationship.

Couple-Oriented Groups

You and your partner can also find support for your relationship by participating in various groups or organizations that encourage committed relationships and healthy interactions. Some couples experience such support through active participation in their children's schools or in their neighborhood—particularly through activities that promote small-group interaction where couples can work and play together. Other couples find support in various social organizations that are oriented specifically to couple- or family-based activities—for example, working in the community food bank together on Saturday mornings or going on weekend camping excursions together.

EXERCISES

EXERCISE 7.1   Identifying Outside Negative Influences

List the major factors outside your relationship—such as intrusions from work, volunteer activity, or other people—that have undermined your relationship. For example:

"I've taken on so much volunteer work that I haven't left enough time and energy for our relationship."

Or

"I never was entirely comfortable with the amount of time we were each going out separately with friends, instead of together. Some of that could be good, but too much pulled us apart as a couple."

For each of the outside factors you listed above that take away from your relationship, describe what you can do, either individually or as a couple, to minimize their effect on your relationship. For example:

"We both value giving back to the community, but we've clearly overdone it. Let's each limit our outside meetings to no more than one night a week."

EXERCISE 7.2 Building On Outside Resources

List the major people and groups you can turn to now or have turned to in the past to support and strengthen your relationship. For example:

"My brother-in-law is someone I admire. I'd like to spend more time with him, not to talk about the affair, but just to be with someone I can learn from and see how he handles various stresses and how he prioritizes his family."

List the groups of people you would like to be part of that would support and strengthen your relationship. For example:

"We're fortunate to live in a family neighborhood with many couples our age. They have lots of informal get-togethers, but we haven't participated very much. Let's start saying yes to those invitations and have some of the families in the neighborhood over to our house."

8

How Could My Partner Have Done This?

Nick was aware that women found him physically attractive. He had a smile and easy manner that others found both comfortable and engaging. It hadn't been that way all along. Always somewhat small for his age, he had been shy and awkward as a teenager. When he finished high school and went to work for his father while most of his friends moved away to attend college, he had felt stupid and inept. But Nick worked hard and gradually built his own construction firm. The shyness he had experienced as an adolescent had now grown into a quiet and sensitive manner that women seemed to find attractive. Still, his lingering self-doubts were never far beneath the surface.

Nick had married Becky soon after she graduated from high school. As years passed, he felt increasing admiration for all she did for their marriage and their children. He had no interest in getting involved with other women and never took flirtation seriously—until Diana came along. She was divorced, and Nick found her a bit intimidating but also quite attractive. So when Diana invited him to lunch to discuss renovations to some rental properties she had bought, he felt both flattered and apprehensive. Diana complimented Nick on all he had accomplished and made it clear that she was attracted to him. He had never been unfaithful to Becky, even though recently she frequently seemed irritated and uninterested in any physical closeness. But when Diana made it clear she wasn't looking for a serious relationship with Nick but only wanted *some physical intimacy with a man she admired, his feelings over-whelmed his logic. For six months he and Diana pursued a sexual relationship, while keeping talk about their personal lives generally off-limits.*

Just as affairs can happen in a good relationship, affairs can "happen" to good people. Good, loving, and previously faithful partners can make bad decisions that lead them astray. When you and your partner first pledged to be faithful to one another, it's unlikely that you imagined you would ever experience this kind of betrayal. You trusted your partner not to hurt you in this way. No matter what disagreements you had, no matter what struggles you experienced, you didn't expect to suffer your partner's affair. Now you need to make sense of how the person you loved and trusted could have done this.

In this chapter, we're going to help the injured partner consider aspects of the involved partner that may have contributed to the affair, a process that is useful even if the involved partner chooses not to do this work. However, if you're the involved partner, we strongly encourage you to read through this chapter to gain a better understanding of yourself and how you came to have an affair. At the very least, please read "A Special Message to the Involved Partner" on pages 168–169.

How did the involved partner choose to get involved? If the affair continued beyond one or two occasions, why did the involved partner persist? If the affair is still going on, why won't they just end it? How you answer these questions will influence how you decide to move on and how well you carry out whatever relationship decisions you make down the road.

It's important to achieve a *balanced* view of your partner. It's unlikely that the person you fell in love with and chose to commit to has no positive qualities, despite having hurt you deeply. If you haven't already decided to end this relationship, then you need to consider if and how you could work to regain a caring and trusting relationship with this person who betrayed you. You won't be able to do this without considering your partner's vulnerabilities that led to an affair and without at least some understanding or compassion. Moreover, if you want your partner to join you in exploring the context that led to the affair, you'll need to challenge and perhaps soften your own perspective to make it safe enough for your partner to engage in this process.

Another reason to pursue a balanced view comes into play if you decide to end this relationship and there are children involved. In that case, it will be important to continue to collaborate as parents. Research consistently affirms that *the most important factor in children's adjustment to divorce is how effectively their parents can work together after ending their relationship.* You and your partner will both find it hard to parent together if either one of you views the other as having no positive or redeeming qualities.

Pursuing a balanced view also requires avoiding the opposite extreme of being unrealistically positive or minimizing your partner's responsibility for the affair. That may feel less distressing in the short term because it might allow you to regain a sense of closeness. But if you don't confront issues regarding your partner now, you're more likely to have lingering doubts that could surface at unexpected moments down the road. By then it will be more difficult to engage in the exploration process we're encouraging you to pursue now.

As you read through this chapter, consider not only vulnerabilities but also potential strengths or positive aspects of your partner that may have contributed to the affair. Think about how it came about, how or why it continued, and how it ended or has failed to end. Not everything we invite you to consider here will be relevant to your situation. Don't rush to conclusions that may turn out to be inaccurate or incomplete. Take your time, consider what you read as possible "explanations" for what has happened, and be sure to fit whatever seems to make sense into the larger overall picture that extends beyond your partner to include contributions from your relationship, the outside world, and perhaps even aspects of yourself.

A Special Message to the Involved Partner

If you're working through this book with your injured partner, we commend your decision to participate in this healing process. Not all involved partners are willing to engage in the difficult process of examining how the affair came about in order to work toward recovery. If for no other reason, we encourage you to stick with this process because it's what your partner needs from you. Examining aspects of yourself that made you vulnerable to having an affair may be particularly difficult. It may be hard to resist responding with "Yes, but . . . ": "Yes, but what about the way our relationship was?" "Yes, but what about everything else that was going on?" "Yes, but what about you?" As well as you can for now, try to trust in the overall process in taking a hard look at that part of the big picture that involves you.

This chapter is also intended to help you sort through your own feelings. In our clinical work, we find that people who have participated in an affair often struggle to make sense of their own behavior. "This just isn't like me; how could I have done this?" In confronting their own feelings of confusion, guilt, or shame, involved partners sometimes resist examining parts of themselves that could help them understand how an affair developed. They may then settle on explanations that are incomplete or inaccurate. For example, they may place too much weight on difficulties in their relationship or on positive qualities of the outside affair person as a reason for the affair and then make poor long-term relationship choices as a consequence. We want to help you avoid those risks.

We also want you to assess any aspects of yourself that contributed to the affair so that you can reduce any risks of another affair in the future. In all likelihood, you've already promised your partner and yourself never to have another affair, so further examination of how the affair came about doesn't feel necessary. But it's also likely that you never planned on having an affair the first time you pledged to be faithful "for better or worse." We don't question your intentions to remain faithful. But we do have concerns about how well you can carry out your intentions if you avoid looking at important aspects of yourself that potentially placed you at risk.

Finally, if you're still involved in an affair or sometimes have difficulty dealing with its being over, you need to understand everything you can about why these feelings are continuing. Reading through this chapter to understand yourself better may help you reach decisions that are best for you and your partner in the long run.

How Could My Partner Have Gotten Involved?

Before you try to answer this question, we want to provide you with a way of thinking about factors that might have contributed to your partner's vulnerability to an affair. Some of these may extend well back in time and involve attitudes and beliefs, anxieties or needs, or other tendencies that were in place before you and your partner ever met. Examples might include unrealistic beliefs about how a relationship is supposed to be, lack of confidence in oneself as an intimate partner, or an inability to withstand long periods of unhappiness or stress without much support or relief. Think of such factors as paving the way for an affair, making it more likely. They don't cause an affair to happen, but they can raise the risk of an affair by increasing vulnerability to it if certain other conditions come along.

Other factors that made the affair more likely to occur may have pre-dated the affair by only weeks or months, such as flirting with someone who was also susceptible to an affair, or developing an emotionally close relationship and spending increasing time alone with someone else. Such behaviors don't inevitably lead to an affair, but they clearly lower safeguards and raise the risks.

Finally, there may be factors that "triggered" the affair either separately or in combination with other conditions—from alcohol or other substance use that lowers inhibitions and clouds judgment, to anger toward a partner that leads to an affair as retaliation, or recent loss or trauma that increases the need for comfort or reassurance.

In most cases, answering the question "How could my partner have gotten involved?" requires thinking of all of these kinds of factors—some long-term, others more recent, and some brief or even coincidental. Understanding your partner's vulnerability to an affair involves adopting the larger view. You need to consider not only who your partner *is*, but also how your partner came to be this way and who they're *likely to be* in the future. Exercise 8.1 will help you consider these factors further.

What Was My Partner Looking For?

Popular myths regarding infidelity suggest that men have affairs to pursue better or more frequent sex and to experience the thrill of seduction and conquest, whereas women have affairs to pursue emotional connection and overcome fears of growing older and becoming less attractive. However, the reasons for affairs are as varied as the individuals having them, and relying upon stereotyped reasons for an affair can lead to simplistic, unhelpful perspectives.

AFFIRMATION OF SELF-WORTH

Anyone may feel neglected or unappreciated at one time or another. But several factors can increase such feelings in a way that prompt a person to seek the kinds of affirmation sometimes provided by an affair. One is long-standing self-doubt. Like Nick, whom we described at the opening of this chapter, some people lack confidence in their attractiveness, social status or prestige, or more general purpose in life, and that lack of confidence may go back to adolescence or even earlier. Unresolved self-doubt, a low tolerance for criticism, and very high needs for affirmation or feeling valued by a partner can sometimes outstrip the capacity of a partner or committed relationship to provide nurturing or approval as frequently as desired. When this happens, the involved partner needs to examine those needs for affirmation and comfort and how they could place unrealistic demands on any relationship.

High needs for affirmation (being told that you're important and of value) can be increased when a couple has reduced opportunities for providing caring and support to one another, such as when a new baby arrives. Your partner's need for affirmation can also soar when some event undermines or shakes their feelings of confidence, connectedness, or stability in life—for example, the loss of a job or other financial setbacks, the death of a parent or close friend, physical health problems, or an unwanted change in physical appearance.

Was your partner vulnerable to the need for reassurance from someone else? If so, have they always needed to be reminded that they're a good or valued person? Were there situations leading up to the affair that intensified these needs or interfered with the needs being met within your own relationship?

AFFIRMATION OF SEXUAL ATTRACTIVENESS AND ADEQUACY

Most of us want to feel desirable and successful as sexual partners. When stresses or external demands interfere with physical intimacy, or when the sexual relationship suffers from specific problems of its own, a partner can become more vulnerable to seeking sexual fulfillment or affirmation through an affair.

Sometimes people also pursue an affair as a way of exploring aspects of their sexuality that they're uncomfortable pursuing in their committed relationship. For example, a partner may become particularly aroused by sexual behaviors that they're uncomfortable pursuing with someone with whom they're also emotionally connected. Or a person may be apprehensive about taking a more assertive or creative sexual role if they anticipate that their partner could view this as an unwanted or threatening change—perhaps thinking that "it's too far out there" or "this doesn't fit my partner's image of me." It's not unusual for someone to feel obligated to behave as they always have in their sexual relationship, even if those patterns of physical intimacy fall short of expectations or wishes.

What can you learn from your history together? Has your partner struggled with concerns about their sexual desirability in the past? Have difficulties in your sexual relationship or stresses on your relationship hampered your sex life? Has your partner expressed dissatisfaction with your sexual relationship in the past, or have discussions about this aspect of your relationship felt awkward or difficult?

EMOTIONAL CONNECTION AND INTIMACY

Sometimes it's the pursuit of emotional intimacy that sparks the affair. Shared secrets—including the secrecy of the affair—may heighten the sense of having a special connection or bond with someone else. The intimacy of an affair often feels similar to the intimacy experienced early in courtship—extended personal conversations uncomplicated by the stress of everyday life, feelings of being cared for in a special way, or special efforts to be together. You may have been drawn to your partner in part because their need for emotional closeness matched or balanced your own. But what started out as a shared emotional bond between the two of you may have increased your partner's vulnerability to an affair if your emotional connection became strained or disrupted.

Intimacy can be complicated. Partners need to be able to pursue emotional connection while also tolerating frustrations and separateness. Affairs can appear to offer intimacy without the inherent challenges and strains of a long-term committed relationship. Or the intimacy or excitement of an affair may seem to make the challenges of a committed but unrewarding relationship more tolerable.

When Joury first met Ahmed, she found his devotion comforting. But over time she occasionally found his dependence a bit suffocating. Ahmed had no close friends other than Joury and resented Joury's desire for separate time for herself. Joury gradually began to pull away from Ahmed to reestablish some independence, but Ahmed's resentment then made it more difficult to get back together to enjoy time as a couple.

Joury met Aaron at a yoga class that met weekly. Aaron had never been married, had lots of male and female friends, and pursued a life full of activities outside of work and home. Soon Joury was leaving work early to be with Aaron before Ahmed came home from work. She found it odd that since beginning her affair with Aaron, she actually seemed to feel less distant and less irritable at home.

How do you view your partner's need for emotional connection? In what ways have these been a source of strength in your relationship, and in what ways have they been a challenge or burden? If you and your partner felt more emotionally intimate earlier in your relationship, what would it take to restore more of those feelings now?

FULFILLMENT OF UNREALISTIC EXPECTATIONS

No relationship—and no partner—is perfect. Maintaining a loving relationship requires that partners accept and value each other for who they are, with all their imperfections. That doesn't mean relinquishing the right to request changes in your partner's behavior, and it doesn't mean giving in to abuse or neglect. But it does mean recognizing that no individual and no relationship will ever satisfy all your needs all the time. Failing to come to grips with this reality will ultimately bring hurt and disappointment to both partners.

Sometimes an affair provides something that's missing in the partners' own relationship. It may be passionate sex, freedom from demands or expectations, time away in exciting or relaxed settings, and so on. The truth is that no committed relationship can compete with an affair on these terms. No long-term, committed relationship can be devoted so exclusively to mutual affirmation and pleasure. Affairs are protected from many of the hassles, pressures, and demands of daily living that inevitably intrude into a long-term relationship. Although most partners recognize this, many still hold on to unrealistic expectations that can get them into trouble. Examples are "If our relationship is really a good one . . . " (or "If you really love me . . . "):

    . . . we won't ever have serious disagreements or arguments.

    . . . you'll never hurt my feelings or disappoint me.

    . . . you'll know how I feel without my having to tell you.

    . . . you'll always be there for me when I need you.

    . . . we'll always place each other as our top priority.

    . . . we'll have frequent and passionate sex.

Similarly, unrealistic expectations or beliefs about affairs can get partners into trouble. Examples include the following:

As long as no one else knows about the affair, no one will get hurt.

Just about everyone has affairs or wants to.

A good affair can make a bad relationship better.

Affairs don't need to be complicated or intrude into other areas of life.

Difficulties in tolerating the inevitable disappointments that occur in a relationship, feelings of entitlement or having a sense that "I deserve better than this," and a lack of understanding about the limitations and frequently painful consequences of infidelity can all raise a partner's vulnerability to becoming involved in an affair. So too can the excitement of seduction and a secretive liaison, the passion of a new "first kiss," and all the other heightened sensations that frequently accompany an affair.

To what extent does your partner become bored with "sameness" and require new experiences and a high level of excitement in life? Do your partner's standards for a "good relationship" seem unattainable? Could the two of you find a better way to deal with each other's imperfections, while continuing to work together toward changes in yourselves and in your relationship?

What Did the Other Person See in My Partner?

The same personal qualities that attracted you to your partner may attract others. They too may find your partner particularly understanding, intelligent, charming, or physically attractive. Your partner may also be more desirable to others if they appear outgoing and comfortable in discussing relationships and intimate feelings. The professional achievements, visibility in the community, or physical attractiveness that you find desirable in your partner may all contribute to their being emotionally or sexually attractive to others.

Does this mean your partner shouldn't work toward success, shouldn't be as warm and caring to others, or should neglect their physical appearance? Of course not! However, it does mean your partner needs to recognize their social "currency" or attractiveness to others, maintain suitable vigilance, and keep relationships with others from approaching the boundaries of inappropriate social, emotional, or physical closeness. It means your partner must recognize flirtation and set limits on this so as not to encourage sexual advances. Similarly, your partner needs to anticipate situations where interactions with someone outside your relationship could promote feelings of closeness that could easily escalate.

What positive qualities place your partner at higher risk for being sought out by someone outside your relationship? What steps would your partner need to take to recognize their attractiveness to others, adopt an appropriate level of vigilance, and set boundaries on interactions with others in order to protect the security of your own relationship?

Why Didn't My Partner Resist?

Regardless of what was going on in or around your own relationship, and regardless of how unhappy your partner was or how vigorously they were pursued by someone else, why didn't your partner resist? Why didn't they "just say no"? Restoring emotional security will require confidence that your partner will continue to say no to an outside relationship when things in your own relationship are at their worst. The following are some factors that may lower someone's resistance to an affair.

PROBLEMS WITH COMMITMENT

It's not unusual for partners to have times when they aren't particularly happy with each other or their relationship but remain faithful based on personal values of responsibility or commitment. However, commitment can be undermined by the intensity or duration of relationship problems or from despair about the relationship ever getting better. Feelings of desperation don't excuse your partner's decision to have an affair, but they may contribute to understanding how the affair developed. Hopelessness about the future of one's relationship can whittle away at commitment and lead people to look elsewhere for comfort or companionship.

You need to assess your partner's capacity for commitment. Commitment means buckling down to work it out, even when things are hard or no fun. Has your partner shown the ability to give their all to you, your relationship, or your family in the past, even when things have been tough? If so, the affair probably doesn't simply reflect an inability to commit. However, if your partner has a history of backing off on things they've agreed to do, putting themselves first, or feeling constrained when they need to follow through with difficult tasks when they don't feel like it, then problems with commitment may be an important contributing factor.

LAPSES IN JUDGMENT

Related to problems with commitment are lapses in judgment—impulsive, mostly unplanned actions that are driven primarily by emotions rather than by careful thought. Some people have an impulsive style that involves mainly focusing on what they want in the moment rather than thinking about long-term consequences. They tend to act before they think and to leap before they look. In addition, lapses in judgment might result from failure to recognize the complex or hidden motives of others. For example, perhaps your partner isn't very good at reading other people and their intentions, or your partner doesn't know their own limits, thinking they can handle risky situations when in reality they can't.

When Mieko's art instructor offered to tutor her at his apartment at night because of "understanding" her struggles as an older student with two young children, she never imagined that he might have anything

*other than honorable intentions. She later was surprised by her instruc-
tor's sexual advances and found herself drawn into kissing and intimate
touching before regaining her composure and putting on the brakes.*

At other times, lapses in judgment relate directly to use of alcohol
or other substances that lower inhibitions. Similarly, impaired judgment
sometimes results from emotional disorders such as bipolar disorder. A
partner's affair doesn't necessarily indicate that they have an emotional
disorder. But if your partner does struggle with an emotional disorder
or with problems of substance abuse, it's important to consider how such
difficulties contribute to lapses in judgment and what steps your partner
could take to lower the risks.

Cole had a passion for life that Lydia found energizing when they first
met. He introduced her to all kinds of things—art films, street racing,
even the occasional rave with ecstasy or ketamine. But Lydia eventually
grew tired of participating in some of the "adventures" that Cole was
drawn to and felt relieved when he suggested doing these on his own so
she could have some quiet time for herself.

When Lydia learned from a mutual friend that Cole had recently
had sex with a woman he had met at an out-of-town concert, her vision
of Cole shattered. Although he showed deep remorse and vowed to be
faithful from then on, Lydia eventually concluded that she could never
again feel secure in their relationship. After months of examining how
his infidelity had come about and becoming clearer about Cole's need
for an adrenaline rush and a tendency for breaking rules that he seemed
unable to change, Lydia decided to end their relationship and move on
separately.

RELUCTANCE TO CONFRONT RELATIONSHIP DIFFICULTIES

When a relationship suffers from significant or enduring problems, the
challenge is to engage your partner in looking at them together and trying to resolve them as well as possible. That can involve the risk of dis-
approval, being held accountable for a major portion of the problems, or
having your concerns ignored and feeling unimportant. When partners
feel unable to express themselves, when they fear that voicing their unhappiness may lead to further arguing, or when they're reluctant to go through

the difficult process of constructive conflict, retreat to another relationship that doesn't seem to have the same level of conflict can seem like a safer alternative.

How able and willing is your partner to express or listen to concerns in your relationship? What would it take for both of you to create a safer and more constructive process for confronting relationship difficulties?

EXPRESSION OF DISCONTENT

Some people have an affair as a way of communicating feelings to a partner that they're having difficulty expressing more directly. The most common example is when an affair serves as a final, desperate plea to the other to "hear" that partner's profound unhappiness and need for change. Sometimes the message isn't as much a plea for collaborative change as an expression of anger. The problem, of course, is that this is a high-stakes game. The message may finally be heard, but sometimes the accompanying damage is so great that healing is impossible.

Less frequently, an affair may serve not as a plea to be heard, but rather as an undisclosed decision to end the relationship. These are sometimes described as "exit" affairs. The involved partner has already reached a decision, consciously or not, to leave the relationship and anticipates that having an affair will provoke the other partner to end it for them.

You need to find out from your partner if they considered leaving your relationship when becoming involved in the affair. If so, have they changed their mind? If the affair was used in part to express their unhappiness, will your partner pledge to express these feelings directly and to seek your engagement in the future, even if they feel pessimistic about the outcome?

How Could My Partner Continue the Affair?

Thalia struggled to understand Dion's yearlong affair. Dion had finally confessed to his involvement after one of their children overheard him on the phone planning another secret rendezvous. "How could you have done it?" Thalia repeatedly asked. Dion's ability to lead a dual life deeply troubled Thalia. The betrayal from the affair was traumatic enough. But how could he continue the affair and then come home and engage with her as though nothing was wrong? The continued deception seemed even worse than the affair.

Thalia's dilemma is a common one. A brief affair ended by the involved partner creates its own trauma. But when a partner continues involvement in an affair, maintaining the outside relationship usually requires repeated lies that compound the trauma further. Elaborate cover stories are constructed to conceal secret meetings. Or the involved partner creates a separate email account or gets a separate phone used solely for exchanges with the outside person. Perhaps most painful of all, the involved person may continue to be emotionally or sexually intimate with their partner as though the outside relationship doesn't even exist. This ability to separate the outside relationship from interactions with the injured partner so completely may seem incomprehensible. "How could they keep up the charade for so long? How can I ever trust them when they lied repeatedly with such ease?"

If your partner engaged in an ongoing affair, understanding both *why* and *how* they continued in that relationship is critical to recovery.

Why Did My Partner Continue?

A variety of factors contribute to why someone may continue an affair once it has developed, but common reasons include these expressed in the following scenarios:

- *Feelings of responsibility to the outside person.* Carmen (the outside person) might have left her long-term partner anyway, but Travis knew she had done so in part because of the yearlong affair Travis had with her. Carmen was utterly alone now, and Travis just didn't feel he could abandon her while she was struggling so much.

- *Positive aspects of the outside relationship.* Kaila found Isaac easy to be with—a caring listener who appreciated her playfulness and could tolerate her occasional moodiness. The playfulness at home had faded away years ago.

■ *Pessimism about improving the committed relationship.* Ruth had expressed her concerns about their relationship to Noah as gently as she knew how, but he dismissed her feelings and told her she was unrealistic. When Ruth suggested couple counseling, Noah replied, "I just don't think we need that." If he wouldn't talk with her, how could things ever get better?

■ *Feelings of entitlement.* Kavi worked two jobs to support their family. He didn't expect Palomi's eternal gratitude, but at least she could show some appreciation and try to be a little more affectionate. He wasn't about to go through life without sex. What did she expect?

Paradoxically, some of the qualities that you value in your partner may have contributed to their continuing the affair. For example, you may have been drawn to your partner in part because of their capacity to form a deep emotional and caring relationship. As hurtful as it may be to consider, it's possible that this quality contributed to a meaningful and intimate relationship with the outside person. Similarly, if your partner is someone you've viewed in the past as being responsible and honorable, it may be this sense of responsibility for the other person that contributed to maintaining the affair—no matter how misguided this may seem. As couple therapists, we've worked with numerous involved partners who have struggled to end an affair, only to be drawn back in when the outside person pleads not being able to live without the involved partner or threatens self-harm.

Of course, there also are reasons for continuing an affair that are less readily understood or forgiven. For example, your partner may have intended to maintain the affair so long as it continued to feel rewarding and the costs related to the affair (such as time, money, or threats to your own relationship) remained low. Or your partner may have continued the affair because they were preparing to end your relationship but weren't yet willing to tell you and deal with the consequences.

Part of what you need to assess is how much your partner struggled internally while continuing the affair. Were there times when your partner considered telling you but didn't want to risk damaging your relationship, perhaps losing it? Did your partner ever consider or actually try ending the relationship with the other person? If you're convinced that your partner maintained the outside relationship "with ease"—that they experienced no guilt, shame, or turmoil from continued deception and betrayal—then you'll likely find it more difficult to reestablish trust and emotional security.

How Did My Partner Continue?

Patrick never could have imagined being unfaithful—it went against everything he believed in. But his relationship with Taylor at times felt unbearable, and his escape into a relationship with Micki offered a different world. He didn't let himself think about his family when he was with Micki, and he didn't allow himself to think of Micki when he was at home.

Beyond asking *why* your partner continued in the affair are questions about *how* your partner did so. How could your partner continue to interact with you as though the affair relationship didn't even exist? To understand this common experience, therapists use the term *compartmentalization*—individuals' ability to take the thoughts, feelings, and behaviors of one situation and literally "shut them off as in a compartment" from their thoughts, feelings, and behaviors in a different situation.

We all engage in compartmentalization to some extent. Think about the last time you and your partner drove to work or some social event following an argument at home with each other or with one of your children. Did you "shelve" the inner turmoil and put on your "happy face" when you walked through the door and greeted others? If your work requires you to be "on stage," interact with others throughout the day, or focus heavily on what you're doing at the moment, do you sometimes put conflict from home (or even anticipated positive activities) aside during the day—literally out of mind so that you address what is happening in the moment?

Whereas being able to compartmentalize is essential in many parts of life, it can be used to maintain maladaptive behavior when it means that problematic behaviors are set aside and not thought about. This same process of compartmentalization is a frequent explanation for how individuals involved in an affair maintain their dual lives. For most involved partners, an affair *does* create inner conflict. It often *is* inconsistent with their values, with how they see themselves, and with their genuine caring for their partner. Compartmentalizing the affair relationship—actually separating off the outside person—when with their partner and shutting out thoughts of their partner when with the outside person is often the only way of emotionally managing the inner conflict. Although it's an unsatisfactory explanation for most injured partners, involved partners in various ways often describe, "I just kept things separate. When I was with you, I was with you. When I was with the other person, I was with that person." Even if you and your partner have previously agreed to a nonmonogamous relationship that allows for involvement with other persons, compartmentalization can still can become problematic when it involves a violation of the boundaries that you've set.

Of course, sometimes no such internal struggle exists—as when the involved partner has limited capacity to experience remorse for hurting others, or has already decided to leave the relationship. If that's the situation you face, deciding whether to work toward restoring your relationship could be more difficult.

Your understanding of how your partner continued the affair will be influenced by how you viewed them prior to the affair. Was your partner someone who generally tried to do the right thing? Who felt bad if your feelings were hurt by something they said or did? If your answer to such questions is "yes" or "most of the time," then *compartmentalization* may in part explain how your partner managed their own emotions while maintaining the affair and keeping it secret from you. And if your partner can compartmentalize in such an important part of life, would they commit to living a more integrated life if you consider staying together?

Why Won't My Partner End It?

If your partner is continuing the affair and doesn't want to end it, then you're likely facing all kinds of difficult decisions. Do you give your partner a deadline and an ultimatum? Do you demand a separation while the affair is going on, or do you file for divorce? Do you "wait it out" and trust that your partner will come to their senses and return to your relationship or hope that the strong emotional pull from the other person will burn itself out? In struggling with such questions, you may want to review material in Chapter 4 on how to respond when the affair is still going on. Your decisions about how to deal with your partner's continued involvement in an affair may depend in part on your understanding of why they're reluctant or unwilling to end it.

Positive Aspects of the Affair Relationship

Affairs often affirm one's desirability and provide relief from life's complications, or escape from conflicts elsewhere in life, including at home. The emotional chaos that often consumes a couple's relationship after an affair becomes known can force involved partners to choose between an affair that feels rewarding and a relationship that feels profoundly distressing, with a partner who is hurt and angry. Choosing the latter requires engaging more discomfort in the short term in the hope that something more valuable can be restored or created in the long term.

Emotional Connection to the Outside Person

If the affair relationship has lasted beyond a brief period, there's a possibility that your partner may have developed a strong emotional connection to the outside person. Early in affairs, unrealistic idealization of the outside person and feelings of infatuation are common. However, when an affair has lasted for months or even years, the outside relationship can mature beyond infatuation to develop into deep caring for the other person. Once such a relationship has developed, it's far more difficult to end the affair. Your partner also may feel responsible for the other person's emotional well-being. We don't expect you to have empathy for the outside person, but it may be important for you to recognize what feelings your involved partner still has for the other person that could be contributing to difficulty in ending the other relationship.

> Sofia was a caretaker by nature. Her husband, Tanner, was a faithful provider but emotionally aloof. Sofia met Justin shortly after his wife died and they had begun volunteering together at their community's hospice program. Sofia felt drawn to Justin not only by his gentle and kind nature, but also because of his obvious deep need for her emotionally. When she and Justin first had sex several months after meeting, she felt deeply connected in a way she hadn't for years.

When Tanner learned of Sofia's affair, he insisted she sever her relationship with Justin immediately. Sofia agreed, but her promise proved difficult to keep. Justin texted her daily, professing how deeply he loved Sofia and needed at least to see her. Sofia consented, and several secret meetings followed. There was no further sex, but Sofia longed for the emotional connection they had, and her aloneness at home felt unbearable.

Pessimism about the Outcome of Your Relationship

Your partner's reluctance to give up the affair may also be influenced by ongoing difficulties in your own relationship and pessimism about things getting better. If long-standing struggles in your relationship contributed to your partner's initial vulnerability to an affair, these conflicts may make it more difficult for either of you to commit to your relationship now. Your partner may also be assessing the future quality of your relationship by predicting from the current emotional turmoil rather than considering previous times in your relationship that were less chaotic and more satisfying.

What hopefulness does your partner express about the ability to move beyond this trauma together? Do they recall times in the past when things were significantly better? Can you communicate your own realistic hopefulness for how you can restore or create a better relationship for both of you?

Inability or Unwillingness to Commit to One Person

Your partner may not want to commit to a monogamous relationship. Or they may be willing to end the sexual aspects of an outside relationship but insist on the right to continue a close relationship with the outside affair person on a nonsexual level. Alternatively, your partner may pledge to an exclusive relationship with you but continue to be vulnerable to outside relationships for any of the reasons we've described above. In addition to evaluating how your partner became involved in the affair in the first place, if the affair is continuing, you'll need to assess your partner's capacity for commitment now and in the future, and what you want moving forward.

Why Can't My Partner Move On?

Once an affair has ended, moving on requires that you and your partner work through the trauma of the affair and collaborate in understanding how it came about. It also requires that eventually you both allow thoughts and feelings about the affair to recede into the background as you work toward the future together. Both you and your partner may have difficulty with any of these steps.

Working through the Trauma

You and your partner may continue to struggle with the challenges described in Part I of this book. Involved partners often recognize how hurt the injured partner continues to be, and their reluctance to engage in discussions about the affair may stem from the chaos of stirring things up all over again. Do you or your partner feel "worn down" by the continued turmoil in your relationship? How can you work together to make discussions about the affair less traumatic for you both?

Your partner may also be wrestling with difficult feelings of their own. For example, they may be struggling with having ended a close emotional connection to the outside person but also recognize how difficult it might be for you to hear those feelings. Other times involved partners wrestle with their own frustrations regarding your relationship as a couple but don't believe they're entitled to express such feelings because of their affair. Sometimes they're wrestling with deep guilt and shame over their own behaviors, which can then make it difficult or painful to discuss the pain they've caused you.

Try talking with your partner about their reluctance to discuss the affair. What's making it difficult?

Understanding How the Affair Came About

Involved partners sometimes find it difficult to explore how an affair came about because they're confused themselves about why the affair happened—"It just happened; that's all I know." Your partner may be reluctant or unable to describe the feelings they were having toward you, your relationship, or the outside person that contributed to the affair.

Ellie felt frustrated when she tried to talk with her partner, Lacey, about the reasons for her affair. "She says she wants to know what drove me to it, but she really doesn't. When I talk about how lonely and desperate I felt, she responds by saying, 'How do you think I feel now?' I know I've hurt her deeply, but trying to talk about what was missing in our relationship just seems to hurt her more."

Your partner's motive for *not* wanting to discuss the affair may be to protect you from further hurt or disappointment. Or your partner may be convinced that everything that can be said has already been said. Think about discussions you and your partner have had about why the affair occurred. Do you seem stuck in going over and over the same questions, mostly getting the same answers? What would you or your partner consider a sign of progress in these discussions?

Moving from Thoughts and Feelings Rooted in the Past

Your partner may be reluctant or find it hard to "forget what happened," just as you may be. They can get stuck ruminating about past actions that were so hurtful to you. Some involved partners believe that an important safeguard against "slipping up" in the future is to remind themselves constantly about how they've "messed up" in the past. You may have initially found your partner's guilt reassuring as a safeguard against future betrayal but subsequently found that your partner's preoccupation with the affair prevents your moving on together. If so, talk with your partner about what you need now in the relationship and how that differs from what you needed after you first learned of the affair. This journey is an ongoing process, and what you each need changes over time. Do whatever you can to make sure neither of you gets stuck somewhere in the process so you can decide about the future in a productive way. How do you want the two of you to move forward, perhaps finding a way to reconnect and even rediscover joy and spontaneity? What are each of you able to contribute to that effort now that you couldn't earlier?

Becky, whose husband Nick we described at the beginning of this chapter, struggled to make sense of Nick's affair. If nothing else, he had always been someone she could count on. In the months after Nick disclosed his affair, he and Becky talked about the distance that had gradually grown between them—both emotionally and physically. Nick was reluctant to complain about any of the shortcomings in their relationship, but Becky eventually persuaded him that she cared less about "fault" for the distance that had developed and more about finding ways to overcome it. Nick had the affair, but Nick and Becky together had created the distance in their relationship.

Nick struggled with his shame over having betrayed Becky and was reluctant to examine any explanations that might make it "easier" to understand because he explicitly did not want it to be "easy" for him. But with Becky's support, he gradually confronted long-standing issues involving his own lingering self-doubts that had their roots back in adolescence. Becky didn't simply "get over" Nick's affair after developing a better understanding of his needs that had contributed to it. But over time and with considerable effort, they rebuilt the closeness they each desired and created safeguards against drifting apart.

Creating a Future Together or Apart

You and your partner won't be able to work toward potentially creating a better future together unless you share at least some hopefulness that such a future is possible. Once the affair has ended, your partner's or your own pessimism may continue to block efforts to work together toward building or restoring a more satisfying relationship. If you find yourself in this position, talk with your partner about why you need to join together in working through the healing process. Talk about the advantages you envision for both of you in working through this together and whatever realistic confidence you have in your ability to do so. If your own pessimism has discouraged your partner from working toward a future together, consider what it would take to challenge your pessimism and promote feelings of hopefulness for both of you.

EXERCISES

If you and your partner are both working through these chapters, do the following exercises separately, but then arrange a time to compare and discuss your responses.

EXERCISE 8.1 Aspects of the Involved Partner Contributing
to the Affair

List the major factors about the involved partner that increased their vulnerability to an affair. Consider both negative and positive characteristics. Which of these characteristics have been present for a long time,
and which ones have developed more recently? What would the involved
partner need to change so that these characteristics no longer pose a
threat to your relationship?

An example from the injured partner:

"Lani is outgoing and a great listener, and the guys at work sometimes
seek her out for relationship advice. But she'll need to set better limits
on those conversations, because they can slip into deeper personal
discussions and cross boundaries."

An example from the involved partner:

"I never felt confident about myself growing up, and I recognize now
how that made me more vulnerable to someone who was showering
me with attention. I need to work on my own self-doubts so I can
stand strong and stay 100% faithful in my relationship."

EXERCISE 8.2 Aspects of the Involved Partner That Help
or Hinder Recovery

Make two lists. First, list characteristics of the involved partner that might
make recovery from the affair difficult or make this person vulnerable to
an affair in the future.

An example from the injured partner:

"Immediately after the affair, Jon promised to work less and devote
more time to our relationship, but lately he's slipped back into old
habits again. I need him to renew his limits on work—otherwise I
can't feel confident he won't become vulnerable all over again."

An example from the involved partner:

"When I see how devastated by my affair Miguel continues to be, I
slip into overwhelming guilt and just want to crawl into a hole. But I
see that my withdrawal just makes it worse for Miguel. I need to find

better ways of tolerating those awful feelings so I can stay engaged and continue to work at repairing our relationship."

Second, list strengths or positive qualities of the involved partner that might help in recovery from the affair or protect you from an affair in the future.

An example from the injured partner:

"One thing I know about Riley is that when she's made a mistake in the past, she's typically accepted responsibility, figured out what needed to change, and then committed herself to making those changes, no matter how difficult."

An example from the involved partner:

"Having an affair was an unbelievably horrible decision. I not only betrayed my partner, but I violated my own values. I can work at restoring my own integrity by doing whatever it takes to rebuild trust in our relationship."

9

What Was My Role?

When Kelly first heard that Matt had been seen having dinner at an upscale restaurant with an ex-girlfriend, she simply didn't believe it. Kelly brought up the rumor with Matt anyway, but he denied it. Two months later, a close friend told Kelly about three different occasions when Matt had been seen having dinner with the same woman. When Kelly confronted Matt with the new information, he finally acknowledged that he had run into his old flame six months earlier, and they had been sexually involved several times since.

Kelly's head had been spinning and her heart pounding ever since. How could she have been so naive and not seen it coming? Sure, they had struggled lately, but she never anticipated it could lead to this. Kelly had been so angry the previous night that she vowed to call a lawyer the next day. But Kelly didn't call an attorney; she didn't know what she wanted. And what did Matt want to do about their relationship now? He said he needed more closeness—but felt pushed away by her. He complained that she never approached him passionately but only criticized him when she thought he had messed up somehow. "You're not being fair," Kelly had told him. "We agreed to push ahead in our careers until we'd have more time for each other in another year or two."

Matt didn't think he could wait a couple of years, and Kelly's vision about how they would rekindle their closeness had now evaporated. Had she been blind? Was she to blame for Matt's affair? Could she get Matt back—and did she even want to try?

Kelly wasn't responsible for Matt's decision to have an affair—no matter how inattentive, tired, or critical she may have been. Matt had a choice about whether to respond to his distress by getting involved with someone else. He could have been clearer with Kelly about how unhappy he felt or asked her what she needed from him so she could be available. He could have suggested they get outside help from a professional counselor. But if Kelly wanted to explore whether they could salvage their relationship, she would need to evaluate her own role in increasing its vulnerability to an affair—just as the two of them had to explore Matt's role and what had been going on in and around their relationship that made things worse. Kelly didn't have to agree with Matt's views about her and their relationship, but she at least needed to understand what his views were.

The main goal of this chapter is to help you, the injured partner, consider what roles you played in your relationship prior to your partner's affair, as well as your roles during and following the affair. The involved partner should also read this chapter, particularly "A Special Message to the Involved Partner" below through page 193, addressing how to support and join you in this process.

The work we're encouraging you to do in this chapter is very difficult. Your partner may have tried to assure you that there was nothing wrong with your relationship, but we're asking you to step back and examine your relationship carefully. Think about what you could have done to make your relationship stronger, knowing what you know now. Were there circumstances that made it difficult for you to be the kind of partner you'd really like to be? If you think you may want to restore your relationship, what would that require of you right now—as well as six months or a year from now?

If just reading these questions brings up all the hurt and anger you felt right after learning of the affair, you may not be ready to do some of this work. It may help to remember that *reasons* for an affair are never *excuses* and that *understanding* your partner's perspective isn't the same as *agreeing* with it. Even if you decide not to stay in this relationship, taking a close look at yourself and understanding yourself better may help you achieve greater intimacy and security in future relationships.

A Special Message to the Involved Partner

As the involved partner who had the affair, you have two critical roles in this part of the recovery process. First, you have unique information that your partner needs and can get only from you. Only you know what may have felt lacking in your relationship or what gradually eroded your feelings of closeness or hopefulness for the future. It's also possible that you were quite happy with your partner and that any vulnerabilities in your relationship weren't the critical factors that led to your affair. But given that the affair occurred and you want to move forward, both of you now need to explore whether your partner contributed to any vulnerabilities in your relationship that could be addressed to make things better moving forward.

Second, you need to recognize that your partner can't pursue this important part of understanding and recovering from the affair unless you make this process emotionally safe. Doing so involves the following:

- Taking responsibility for your affair, regardless of what was going on in or around your relationship

- Emphasizing that the goal of exploring your partner's role isn't to assign blame but to clarify what it would now take to build a better, stronger relationship together

- Being sensitive to your partner's deep hurt and expressing your own views in language that doesn't attack or overwhelm your partner

- Being patient when your partner initially responds in an angry or defensive manner and waiting for another time to continue your conversations

In our experience, involved partners can impede this phase of the recovery process by going to one of two extremes: (1) blaming the injured partner or the relationship to excuse their own role or (2) not considering the injured partner's role at all, either because they're afraid it will just hurt the injured partner further or because they don't want to be seen as avoiding responsibility or shifting the blame. However, if you won't consider the possibility of improvement or you're unwilling to take on the work of making things better, your relationship *can't and won't* get better. As couple therapists, we've seen that **relationship traumas such as affairs can often promote important changes in both partners that may not have been possible before if both partners do this stage of the work well**.

If you're willing to explore the injured partner's role in your relationship but your partner isn't, talk with your partner about why this is important to you and emphasize what you hope will come from this process for both of you. If your partner isn't yet ready to explore the questions in this chapter, express your willingness to wait as well as your hope that you can do this together in the near future. Then read through this chapter on your own.

Was the Affair My Fault?

You're not to blame for your partner's affair. But could you have contributed to putting your relationship at risk of infidelity? Perhaps. Whether your goal at this moment is to stay in this relationship or to ensure that you're not vulnerable to the same trauma in any future relationship, you need to consider what you bring to a relationship that may prevent it from working as well as you'd like. As you read the following pages and work through Exercise 9.1, think about the ways in which injured partners sometimes make their relationship more vulnerable to an affair, including the following obstacles:

- Difficulties in meeting your partner's needs for intimacy or for personal growth
- Unrealistic expectations or demands
- Negative behaviors that were too frequent or intense
- Difficulty recovering from relationship disappointments or conflicts
- Difficulty dealing with differences in styles of thinking and feeling
- Reluctance to work on your own contributions to relationship difficulties

Did I Fail to Meet My Partner's Needs?

You can't possibly fulfill all of your partner's wishes or desires; that's not your role. All you can hope for is that you'll strive to meet each other's needs as well as possible to care for one another and nurture your relationship. In

Chapter 6 we described a number of qualities that are important to most couples—emotional connection, physical intimacy, and opportunities for personal growth and fulfillment. Knowing what you know now about your partner and about how healthy couple relationships work, are there ways you could have made yours better?

Consider your emotional relationship. How important have emotional connection and intimacy been to you and your partner in the past? Think back to times when your partner may have wanted simply to relax or play together but you thought it was more important to get some work done. Did you share responsibility for creating opportunities to be together? Was physical intimacy lacking in your relationship? Did your partner prefer a different kind of physical intimacy than you did, such as more nonsexual touching like hugging or holding hands? Consider also your partner's needs to grow as an individual. Did you listen to your partner's frustrations and dreams, supporting your partner in good times and bad? If despite your best intentions and efforts, you sometimes fell short in fostering intimacy and personal growth, what can you do differently in the future?

> After Alana's mother died, an emptiness washed over her that she couldn't shake; her children were off having families of their own, and her husband, Carlos, seemed absorbed in managing his thriving business. Carlos recognized that Alana was struggling, but he wasn't sure how to respond. Alana had always been fiercely independent. He would never have expected her to feel desperate enough to succumb to an affair.

Did I Drive My Partner Away?

You didn't drive your partner into having an affair. But you may have contributed to hurtful exchanges or permitted stressors from the outside to have a destructive impact on your relationship. How would your partner describe your approach to dealing with differences between the two of you? Think of times when your partner was clearly upset; were you able to acknowledge their feelings without emphasizing your own complaints? Or when your own feelings were hurt, were you able to express these constructively? Separate from any disagreements, did you both do what was needed to protect your relationship from outside stressors? Try to identify what you would need to do differently now to keep outside influences from putting your relationship at higher risk.

What expectations of your own did you bring into your relationship? Although having high expectations for your family can be a good thing, *excessive* expectations or demands can fuel resentment or cause your partner to believe that whatever they do will never be good enough. How did you convey your own needs and desires, and did your partner feel able to meet these at least most of the time?

> Alexa and Logan had known each other since the seventh grade and married two years after they graduated college, but then their paths started to diverge. She entered veterinary school, while he took over a portion of his family's farm. Alexa was disappointed that Logan lacked ambition and seemed content to live out a quiet, modest life as his parents had. She wanted more for them and encouraged Logan to pursue partnerships in neighboring farms that were becoming available. The more she pushed, the deeper he dug in. When Alexa's work responsibilities kept her out late at night and Logan noticed that she seemed more distant during infrequent sex, Logan felt progressively less desired and less valued. Within a year, he pursued an affair with a woman he had known in high school.

What Did the Outside Person Have That I Don't?

There may be a variety of things that the outside affair person had that you don't, but we want to be clear about one that stands out above all the rest: *The outside affair person had the luxury of interacting with your partner in a relationship that was likely devoted exclusively to mutual pleasure, without all the additional responsibilities and intrusions that confront a long-term couple relationship.* This, more than anything else, defines the fundamental difference between an affair and a committed relationship. It also accounts for why you can't compete in the same ways with an affair partner. You have different roles. We want to make sure that neither you nor your partner compares you with the outside person in ways that are simply unrealistic and unfair.

Of course, the other person may have characteristics that your partner values and that you will never have. For example, you can't change your age. You can't choose your body type, and there may be limits to your influence over your own health or other physical characteristics. You may not be able to match either the career status or the income of the outside person. You may not be able to achieve the same flexibility in your schedule or freedom from competing responsibilities. You may not always be able to look your best, put on a happy face, avoid difficult topics, express admiration for your partner, or create separate space when either you or your partner feels pressured.

By their very nature, affairs differ so dramatically from committed couple relationships that comparing the two to determine which seems better in the long run isn't realistic. Similarly, the roles of an outside affair person and a partner in a long-term committed relationship are so different that comparing yourself (or your partner) with the outside person is neither realistic nor productive.

How Should I Work to Be Different?

There's probably none of us who couldn't be a better partner by being more conscientious, more patient, more attentive, or more understanding. The goal in examining your contributions to your relationship is to engage in thoughtful reflection on what you value, how you believe loving partners can best care for each other, and carefully assess how you could come closer to being the kind of loving partner you aspire to be. Listen to your partner's concerns about your relationship and include their perspective in your assessment of yourself—but also examine your own vision for how good relationships work and what this requires on your part.

Understanding your own relationship patterns as they've developed over your lifetime may offer you a different perspective on what you'd like to keep doing in your current relationship and what you'd want to change. For example, how did you develop your own ways of dealing with difficult feelings, communicating your needs, and connecting emotionally or physically? How did your parents express their feelings toward each other and resolve conflicts or reach decisions together? Did members of your family generally "do their own thing" independently of one another? Recognizing the patterns in your past can give you more control over what you decide to do in the future.

Finally, be sure to keep in mind the principle of balance. Any personal characteristic, taken to the extreme, may not serve you or your relationship well. For example, perhaps your enduring optimism prevented you from recognizing important problems emerging in your relationship. Or your strong work ethic or deep sense of responsibility to others may at times have left you with little physical or emotional energy for your partner and your own relationship. When deciding how to work toward being a better partner, consider both your shortcomings and your strengths and how to use these strengths more effectively for your relationship.

> After learning of Jillian's affair, Connor was reeling in shock and anger. He didn't want to lose Jillian, and she claimed she didn't want to lose Connor, either. But she described drifting so far apart that she had felt as though she was drowning without a lifeline and that Connor had simply turned away. Connor and Jillian both worked 12-hour days, sometimes for weeks on end. They thrived on challenges and made a good team. But over the last year, things had changed. Connor vaguely recalled Jillian complaining about feeling stuck in her own career and resentful of long hours with little advancement and then being upset when Connor worked during weekends at home.
>
> Jillian didn't blame Connor for her affair, and regretted her decision more deeply than she could ever express. She begged Connor to forgive her and also to work with her to make things right. Connor recognized that, for both of them, the changes would require more than minor adjustments. If he wanted their relationship to work, they'd both have to restructure their lives in some major ways. Connor hadn't run from challenges in the past, and he wasn't about to run from this one.

Should I Have Seen It Coming?

Intimate relationships are built in part on trust. One reason that learning of a partner's affair feels so traumatic is that frequently it's totally unexpected. You may be crying out now, "How could I have been so foolish to trust my partner? How could I have been so stupid?" There's nothing foolish or stupid about having trust. Trust in a couple's relationship is more than a good thing—it's essential to security and emotional intimacy.

At the same time, you may have failed to detect clear signals regarding your partner's possible unhappiness or wavering commitment. We're not talking here about evidence you might have uncovered if you'd been more suspicious and taken on the role of a detective. Instead, we're talking specifically about situations in which partners have expressed deep disillusionment, have made statements about ending the relationship, or have otherwise demonstrated disregard for important expectations in your relationship. The question to ask yourself isn't "Could I have known about the affair earlier if I had been more suspicious?" but instead "Were there clear signs that I could have responded to earlier to improve our relationship or address concerns?" There might have been indicators specifically suggesting a possible affair; alternatively, you might have missed signals about overall distress that needed to be addressed, even if you would not have predicted that those foretold a possible affair.

Such clear signs might include, for example, your partner no longer inviting you to social events you had previously attended together—to separate you from the outside affair person or from others who may know of the affair. Some people stop providing information about how they can be reached when away—whether for the evening or when out of town. Were there other signs you may have missed or ignored? Did your partner express unhappiness and try to get you to talk about this? Did you notice withdrawal from physical connection—for example, pulling away from your touches or no longer showing an interest in sexual intimacy? If you can now see that the signs were there, consider what it was about yourself that might have made it more difficult to recognize or discuss these. For example, perhaps your partner's unhappiness made you too nervous to talk about the issues directly, or perhaps you underestimated the problems or hoped they would pass with time.

Knowing what you know now, take some time to reflect on what it would require for you to be vigilant in a healthy way—not unduly suspicious and mistrustful—but alert to early signs of relationship problems that you could address with your partner.

Could I Have Stopped It?

If someone is determined to have an affair, there's probably little that their partner can do to prevent it. Just as you weren't responsible for your partner's affair, you may not have been able to stop it once it occurred. However, there may have been things that you did or didn't do that made the affair easier to begin, easier to continue, or more difficult to stop.

Did I Set Too Few Limits?

Healthy relationships have boundaries—places where you and your partner both put up a stop sign, and neither of you goes beyond that point. Such boundaries involve expectations about how you interact with each other and with those outside your relationship, including friends and coworkers. A relationship can become more vulnerable to an affair when expectations regarding boundaries aren't made clear or when violations are minimized or ignored. It's possible to become too accommodating to your partner's behaviors that cross the line—for example, ignoring flirtatious exchanges with another person. When your partner starts to go beyond the boundaries and doesn't take personal responsibility for ending such violations, it's important for you to step in, express concern, and help to reestablish the boundaries collaboratively.

People sometimes fail to realize how important such limits are if they grew up in families lacking appropriate boundaries. Were the boundaries between members of your family and outsiders clear and appropriate? Do you recall ever seeing either of your parents express too much affection toward other people? Or perhaps you can remember times they divulged too many details about personal or family matters to others. It's mainly within families that individuals learn where to set boundaries. If loose or poor boundaries were all you experienced, it might be difficult for you to know where to set healthy boundaries in your own relationship. On the flip side, if you experienced past relationships that had overly strict or even controlling kinds of boundaries (for example, an ex-boyfriend who insisted that you never hang out with any of your friends unless he was there with you), you may initially struggle to identify what healthy boundaries look like in your own relationship.

It may also be that the boundaries you and your partner mutually agreed to are intentionally more flexible and "open" than those in more traditional, monogamous relationships. If so, that may mean that you can't necessarily talk about your relationship concerns with friends or family who may not be comfortable with or agree with your relationship boundaries.

Peyton and Jules's relationship grew over several months from a close friendship to an intimate partnership. Each of them retained close friendships with other women, some of whom they had been involved with intimately. When Jules began going out with one of those women on nights that Peyton had to work, Peyton tried not to feel jealous. She and Jules had agreed that separate emotional relationships with other women were "okay" but sex was not. Later, when Jules shared that she had resumed a sexual relationship with her friend, Peyton felt deeply wounded but also wondered if she was just being "too old-fashioned."

When you and your partner experiment with boundaries in interacting with others, it can be hard to know what will work and what will feel okay, and whether it will feel consistent with your core values. The important thing is to be honest with yourself and your partner about your feelings as both of you interact with others. Jealousy signals feelings of threat to your relationship; someone else seems to be getting what you want to remain just between the two of you. Paying attention to feelings of jealousy is important—not because jealousy is bad, but so that you can recognize and reflect on it and then decide whether the situation that sparked the jealousy is an actual threat to your relationship, or you're still comfortable with prior boundary decisions, or the jealousy is just a temporary feeling that you expect to decrease with time. Feelings of jealousy are important to notice no matter how you've defined your relationship in terms of boundaries that are to be respected.

Or you may know what appropriate boundaries look like for you and your relationship but didn't know what to do when you first noticed them being crossed. Many people deny or minimize the early warning signs of an affair because these signs make them so uncomfortable. Talking about those signs brings them out in the open and makes them more real. You might have worried that bringing up your concerns would drive your partner into the outside relationship you suspected was developing. Or perhaps you feared being labeled "overly jealous" or so insecure that you couldn't let your partner have any friends.

Avoiding difficult discussions about relationship boundaries can reduce discomfort in the short run, but such avoidance can make the relationship more vulnerable to an affair in the long run. Did you and your partner have clear agreements regarding emotionally intimate, flirtatious, or sexual interactions with others? If you observed times when your partner's behavior appeared inconsistent with such agreements, did you raise this concern directly in a nonattacking way?

> Carla didn't like the way Jabari joked with other women. When she told him how she felt, he called her "uptight," and she privately wondered whether he was right. She had often felt awkward socially, and Jabari's flirty charm was one of the qualities she had found attractive at first. Now it made her nervous, but she kept quiet because whenever she challenged him, he laughed at her and told her to "chill." Later, after learning of Jabari's affair, Carla felt like a fool. Why hadn't she listened to her instincts? She wouldn't put up with that kind of disrespect again.

Even though you now know that your partner engaged in an affair, you might still be tempted to look the other way if you see signs suggesting the affair is continuing or a new one may be starting. There are all kinds of reasons that people decide not to confront an ongoing affair—to try to hold on to their relationship or maintain a belief that "everything's fine," preserve their own self-esteem, shelter their children from learning of the involved partner's infidelity, or maintain the facade of "a happy couple" with friends and family. If your partner is continuing interactions with an outside affair person, review Chapter 4 to remind yourself of how to construct boundaries that will protect you and your relationship.

Did I Contribute to Interactions That Made the Affair More Tempting?

This is a tricky question to ask yourself. It's almost inevitable that your interactions with your partner will be intensely negative right after the affair has been revealed. But if severely negative interactions continue for months or longer, your partner may decide that your relationship can't be salvaged despite any efforts on their part. When your partner has recently had an affair, it's not reasonable to insist that you relinquish any hurt or anger and focus only on positive interactions. But when smoldering resentment, hostile interactions, or disengagement persist for too long, either partner may become so discouraged and hopeless that there's little motivation for working on the relationship. Unfortunately, a person who's had an affair might resume involvement with the outside person to escape from the hurt and anger of the injured partner or because they're missing feelings of connection. Such a decision is the responsibility of the involved partner and obviously isn't a healthy decision for your relationship; we're only encouraging you to consider how your own actions influence, but don't cause, your partner's choices.

> When Mandy discovered Trent's affair, she was furious and determined to make Trent hurt as much as she did. She told him to move out of the house and, when he gave her a startled look, she insisted he sleep on a mattress thrown on the floor of the family room. When their teenage children asked what was going on, she told them everything she knew about their father's affair. She also soon told her own family and made sure Trent's family knew about his affair as well. Mandy suspended standing engagements with their couple friends, explaining that Trent had "become involved with someone else." Within a week, Trent had virtually no one to talk to and few places he could go without embarrassment.
>
> Trent ended his affair and informed Mandy of this, but over the next two months it made no difference. Mandy barely acknowledged him when they were together in the house and announced she had consulted an attorney. Trent had long since given up on having dinners with the family, instead staying at work after hours and picking up a sandwich before heading home. When the outside person sent him a brief text one afternoon asking him if he was okay, he responded with how miserable he was—and several weeks later their affair resumed.

Like his decision to start the affair, Trent alone was responsible for the decision to rekindle it. But Mandy's hurt and anger may have blinded her to the fact that her response gave Trent little hope of salvaging their relationship—even though a part of her still wished for that outcome. If you want your relationship to have at least a chance to recover—even if you're uncertain right now whether that's what you want in the long term—think about how frequently and how intensely you express your hurt and anger to your partner or avoid your partner. How could you temporarily step back to help yourself regain control of your feelings? How do fear and profound sadness overwhelm your ability to interact with your partner more constructively? It's natural to feel deeply hurt, anxious, or angry after learning of a partner's affair, but ultimately it's important to find more effective ways to deal with these feelings if you think you may want your relationship to continue.

Are My Actions Making Recovery More Difficult?

Intense negativity and the absence of positive interactions can make it more difficult for either of you to recover long after an affair is over. If your partner's affair has ended but you seem stuck in angry exchanges, cycling over and over through the same painful discussions without gaining any headway or relief, it's important to figure out how to try to move forward. Likewise, if you've mostly withdrawn from your partner, eventually changes will be needed if you want to consider staying together. Maybe your partner is continuing to behave in ways that threaten the security of your relationship. Or perhaps other unresolved issues are keeping you and your partner in heightened conflict. However, it's also possible that what's going on with *you* is making recovery more difficult for either you or your partner. It's important to explore whether that's the case and, if so, how you could manage things differently. Exercise 9.2 will help you do this.

What's Making This More Difficult for Me Now?

Above and beyond the traumatic impact of a partner's affair, there may be aspects of yourself that make the initial devastation even worse than it might be otherwise or more difficult to recover from in the weeks or months that follow. Understanding these aspects better may help you in your own recovery and may also help your partner be more patient as you struggle to get through this.

FEAR OF VULNERABILITY

You may be finding recovery especially difficult because at some level you're still reeling from shock. The more trusting you were of your partner prior to the affair, or the harder it seemed to even *imagine* the possibility of your partner's being unfaithful, the more profound the trauma of learning about the affair is likely to have been. *Recovery requires moving from exclaiming "I can't believe it" to declaring "I need to understand it."*

The trauma of an affair can also be worse if it reopens old wounds. These injuries might have occurred earlier in this relationship, in previous relationships, or even in the family in which you grew up. Repeated betrayals, even those experienced in different relationships, can magnify the intensity of your hurt and leave you struggling with the terror of allowing yourself to become vulnerable once again. The only way to remain safe for sure is to remain emotionally distant—either through conflict or by withdrawal. By contrast, rebuilding trust requires accepting risk; restoring intimacy demands your vulnerability. If one of the barriers to restoring closeness now involves betrayals from long ago, let your partner know this. Doing so may help both of you place the affair in a larger context in ways that allow you to be less reactive to each other.

MORAL CONVICTION

Strong values are generally good for both individuals and relationships. When your partner violates a core value such as commitment to emotional and sexual fidelity, it can be difficult to piece together positive and negative qualities of your partner into a complete picture that makes sense. Sometimes a person whose partner had an affair will say, "I swore that I would never stay in a relationship with someone who cheated on me. To go back on that now would mean violating my own values." The problem with this stance is that sometimes situations like an affair relate to multiple values that don't necessarily lead to the same conclusion. For example, you might struggle with how to pull together your competing values affirming the importance of sexual fidelity and those affirming the importance of confronting relationship challenges and working toward reconciliation.

We don't presume to tell you what values you should have or what priorities you should give them. But we do encourage you to consider how you reach decisions when they involve multiple and perhaps conflicting values. If you value repair and recovery in intimate relationships, how can you include that value in decisions you're wrestling with now about you and your partner?

PRIDE AND INFLUENCE FROM OTHERS

No one wants to appear foolish. Deciding to work toward recovery in a relationship following a partner's affair is hard enough—but it can be even more difficult if other persons convey that doing so is "weak," "foolish," or "a big mistake." Working toward an informed decision about how best to respond to your partner's affair and whether to stay in your relationship— regardless of what decision you eventually reach—is neither foolish nor unhealthy. You shouldn't end your relationship to avoid appearing weak any more than you should continue it to appear strong. How you appear to others isn't nearly as important as what's best for you in terms of your own long-term happiness and well-being. Be sure the decisions you reach are based on your own careful assessment of your partner, your relationship, your children's needs, and yourself—not on the opinions of your extended family, your friends or, least of all, people with their own axes to grind and their own interests at heart. Perspectives from people you value and respect might provide valuable information, but ultimately your decision has to be right for you.

Am I Making This More Difficult for My Partner?

Your partner may be struggling with their own thoughts and feelings about the affair, how it came about, and what's happened since. You can't resolve your partner's struggles, and it's not your responsibility to make the aftermath easier for your partner, but you can avoid making your partner's recovery more difficult—not only for their sake but for yours and your relationship's sake.

NOT CONTAINING YOUR EMOTIONS

As time goes on, it's important that you learn how to care for yourself and find ways to calm yourself when negative feelings threaten to get out of control. Repeatedly asking the same questions about the affair or having the same arguments, with the same intense feelings and without any progress, can eventually wear your partner out as well as you. That doesn't mean your partner doesn't have a responsibility to engage with you in discussions about how or why the affair happened or what the implications are now. But it does mean that you're both responsible for *how* you engage in these discussions and how often.

When someone hurts you deeply, it's common to want to hurt them back—but deliberately punishing your partner or withholding any forms of positive interaction needs to decrease and eventually come to an end. We don't believe you should become physically or sexually intimate before you're emotionally ready—but when emotional or physical distance is used to punish or get even, such distancing behaviors can become destructive. Similarly, refusing to engage in warm or even casual discussions, rejecting genuine acts of caring from your partner, or avoiding opportunities for positive interactions of any kind may serve to express your anger or protect you from feeling vulnerable in the short run but jeopardize the possibility of restoring your relationship in the long run. You and your partner both need to have healthy reasons to believe that your relationship has the potential to feel good again.

UNDERMINING YOUR PARTNER'S RELATIONSHIPS WITH OTHERS

You and your partner will likely continue to have times when significant conflict or emotional distance comes between you. During these times, it's important that your partner have *appropriate* sources of compassion and emotional support. It's important that you promote your partner's relationships with your children, extended family, or good friends who support your relationship. Speaking in harsh, critical ways about your partner to others who have offered caring to your partner in the past risks undermining valuable support for your partner in moving past the affair and engaging in difficult relationship work with you now.

FAILING TO RECONCILE YOURSELF TO UNCERTAINTY

Injured partners' need to understand the affair to the point where it "makes sense" usually stems from a belief that if they understood the partner's affair completely, they might be able to prevent it from happening again or would no longer struggle with why it happened. But even after you and your partner explore all the contributing factors to the best of your ability, the affair may never make sense to either of you. At some point, virtually everything that could possibly have contributed to your partner's affair will have been discussed. Beyond that point, continued "rehashing" of the same material is unproductive. It doesn't help you feel more secure, and it can erode hope that your partner may have that the two of you can ever get beyond the affair.

Can you resign yourself to never *completely* understanding how your partner came to engage in an affair? You'll never fully understand why your partner had an affair because your partner could have chosen the alternative path *not* to have the affair. Can you move on to rebuild trust and intimacy knowing that you can never be absolutely certain that another affair couldn't happen? What are the potential costs to you and to your relationship if you can't find a way to do that?

Can I Keep an Affair from Happening Again?

If your partner becomes determined to have another affair, there's really nothing you can do to prevent it. But you *may* be able to reduce the likelihood that your partner will have another affair. You can challenge your partner to deal with their own personal characteristics that increased their risk for engaging in an affair. You quite possibly can change your own contributions to conflict, emotional or physical distance, or susceptibility to outside stressors that increased the risk of an affair. And you can examine any aspects of yourself that currently may be making recovery for yourself or your partner more difficult and then work to change these. You both might need to change how you interact with others or navigate a difficult environment you live in. None of these will guarantee that another affair couldn't occur in the future, but together they may substantially lower the risk.

All of these efforts on your part will require a degree of trust. By definition, *trust* means not knowing for sure and moving forward in the face of that uncertainty. The trust you need to have now if you decide to stay in your relationship is neither absolute nor blind. Rather, it's a measured trust that reflects your understanding of potential contributing risk factors and whatever evidence you have of your partner's commitment to rebuild a relationship in which mutual caring, respect, and faithfulness guide partners' behaviors every day. Reaching an informed decision about whether you and your partner can achieve this will require you to pull together all you've learned so far in Part II of this book.

> Kelly, described at the beginning of this chapter, at first found it difficult to consider her own role in their relationship before Matt's affair. However, as she gradually gained better control of her own feelings and her intense anger at Matt waned, she began to notice his efforts to be more involved at home, to hear her deep hurt, and to respond to her needs. Matt ended his affair within a week after Kelly learned of it. He stopped blaming Kelly for problems in their relationship but also avoided talking with her about their relationship at all. At first Kelly felt relieved when Matt no longer pointed to his unhappiness in their relationship as a reason for his affair, but eventually his silence turned into her concern that they hadn't really fixed anything.
>
> A turning point came one night when Kelly approached Matt and said she was still deeply hurt by his affair but was even more fearful that this could destroy their relationship if they didn't find a way to learn from it. After trying unsuccessfully to get Matt to discuss his unhappiness that contributed to his affair, Kelly finally exclaimed, "Look—at this point I'm less concerned about assigning blame than I am with getting this right. We just can't go on this way—with me worrying that you're too unhappy to stay, and you worrying that I'm too hurt or angry to move on. We won't even have a chance unless we're both willing to talk and listen. I need you to trust that I'm ready to do both."
>
> Their recovery wasn't easy and required many difficult discussions. The challenges of balancing the needs of their relationship with the pressures of their respective careers at times seemed overwhelming. But struggling with these challenges together began to produce greater understanding and closeness, in contrast to the distance they had both felt previously.

EXERCISES

If you and your partner are both working through these chapters, do the following exercises separately, but then arrange a time to compare and discuss your responses.

EXERCISE 9.1 Aspects of the Injured Partner Contributing to Vulnerability to an Affair

This exercise has two parts. First, look back at your relationship prior to the affair. To the extent that it fits, make a list of ways that the injured partner (1) wasn't meeting important needs of the person who had the affair, or (2) wasn't doing what they realistically could to make the relationship work.

An example from the injured partner:

"I have to admit that as I got busier at work, when I came home I wasn't fully present. I was so caught up in dealing with my own issues that I didn't take time to hear about his day. That doesn't excuse his affair. But I can see how he might have been drawn to someone who seemed more eager to listen."

An example from the involved partner:

"Melissa is emotionally intense—it's one of the things that drew me to her. But whenever she was frustrated—whether with me or anyone else—her reactions were just too much for me. I found myself always on edge and wanting to escape."

Now look back to the time when the relationship with the outside person was developing or the affair was taking place. List factors that may have made it hard for the injured partner to recognize that an inappropriate relationship was developing or more difficult to demand that the affair come to an end.

For example, the injured partner might now realize:

"I've always been reluctant to stand up for myself. I was afraid that if I confronted my partner with my suspicions about the affair, somehow I'd look stupid or my partner wouldn't even respond—so I just kept quiet for too long."

Or, the involved partner might realize:

"I think he loved me so much that he just couldn't allow himself to see that my 'friendship' with the other person wasn't just a friendship. His wish to keep the dream of our relationship alive made him deny what was happening, and then we just couldn't talk about it."

EXERCISE 9.2 Aspects of the Injured Partner That Help or Hinder Recovery

This exercise also has two parts. First, list things that the injured partner is doing or aspects of that person that make it more difficult for either person to recover from the affair.

An example from the injured partner:

> "I just hate the conflict it causes when I say what I need to say or ask the questions I need to ask. There's so much we really need to understand if we're going to get beyond this, but I can't get myself to bring it up. If we don't find a way to discuss the affair in more detail, I'm afraid I may stay silent and miserable forever."

An example from the involved partner:

> "I know Brandon, and anytime he's been hurt, he wants to strike back. He doesn't typically move on until he's had his revenge. I know I've hurt him badly, and I want to do whatever I can to get us back on track. But when he continues to attack me over and over, it just drives the wedge between us even deeper."

Now list strengths or positive qualities of the injured partner that might help in recovery from the affair.

An example from the injured partner:

> "Even when I've been hurt badly by someone, if I see that we can make things work, I'm able to do whatever work is needed to repair things. I try to learn from the past, not live in it."

An example from the involved partner:

> "Although the distance between us feels really painful, I appreciate how Sonia's hanging in there and trying to hold us together as a family. She still initiates our family outings and looks for ways to encourage my involvement with the children. That takes real character."

10

How Do I Make Sense of It All?

"Making sense of it all" is less about *why* the affair occurred and more about *how* it happened. How did your relationship or your partner become vulnerable? What went wrong, or what failed to go right? What would have to happen now to restore confidence and security in your relationship, and are those changes possible or realistic? If you've worked through Chapters 6 through 9, you've already accomplished much of the work to answer these questions. Nevertheless, it may have been difficult to pull all the pieces together in a way that allows you to see the big picture. In this chapter we'll guide you through the process of reviewing the work you've already done, pulling out the most important insights you've gained, and using these to construct a coherent narrative or story of the affair.

How Do I Sort Through Everything I've Learned?

The first step is to review the work you completed in previous chapters. If you haven't yet completed the exercises for Chapters 6 through 9, work through those now. Exploring the full range of influences that could have contributed to this affair is critical to identifying what's most important in understanding how these influences interacted with each other.

Ideally, you and your partner have each worked through these exercises and have already discussed your responses. If not, it's not too late to encourage your partner to join you in this effort. If working through the previous chapters separately has been helpful to you in interacting more positively with your partner, discuss these changes with your partner and describe how things could be even better if your partner would join you in the process. If you haven't already done so, ask your partner to read the first part of Chapter 6 describing why engaging in this process together is so important to you. If your partner hasn't been working through this book with you but agrees to try it now, be patient as your partner works to catch up with you. Go slowly, taking one chapter at a time, discussing your perspectives and trying to build some common ground before going on to the next one.

Then—whether separately or with your partner—review your responses to each of the exercises. From everything you've learned, try to highlight the most important factors you've identified that contributed to your relationship being at risk. Sometimes people overlook important factors when first working through a chapter but recognize such factors more clearly after working through subsequent chapters. After you've reviewed your responses to each of the preceding four chapters and have highlighted the most important contributing factors that you've identified, try to sort these into the following three categories:

- Negative influences and stressors that placed your relationship at risk (for example, high levels of conflict or feeling emotionally or physically disconnected)

- Positive qualities that contributed to increased risk (for example, leadership skills resulting in too many outside commitments)

- Absence of adequate protective factors (for example, not creating enough opportunities for positive interactions between the two of you or lack of involvement in social groups or activities that support your relationship)

Then, within each of these categories, divide these factors into two groups based on when they were most important: (1) before the affair or (2) during or after the affair. A little later in this chapter, we'll show you how one couple introduced in Chapter 8—Nick and Becky—completed a worksheet to pull together their understanding of what happened in their own relationship.

How do you determine what's most important? There's no simple answer to this essential question. What appears insignificant to one partner can seem vitally important to the other. For example, conflicts with the children may have occurred more frequently or had greater impact for one parent than the other, or one partner may have felt more stressed by financial concerns than the other. It's not essential that you and your partner agree completely on every factor you identify as contributing to vulnerability to an affair. It *is* important that there be substantial overlap in your perspectives and that each of you acknowledge and find a way to respect the other's viewpoint, even if you might see it differently.

How Do I Pull the Pieces Together into a Coherent Picture?

Developing a coherent picture of the affair is like filming a movie with a wide-angle lens or zooming out in the view. You need to zoom out or use a wide-angle lens to make sure everything that's relevant shows up on the screen; using too narrow a lens or zooming in too tightly leaves out some important details entirely and leaves other details out of focus and distorted. You also need a wide-angle lens to see how the different characters and forces interact and influence each other. Watching a character jump off a bridge may not make sense until you see the wider view that shows a car careening wildly toward that person after one of the tires blows out.

Similarly, a meaningful understanding of the affair is more like a movie than a photograph. You need to know how things developed over time, not just at one particular point such as when the affair began. In short, the narrative or story you develop for the affair needs to have a beginning, a middle, and—we hope—an end. The various factors to consider in developing your narrative are summarized in the box on page 214.

In Chapter 8, you read about Nick and Becky and learned about Nick's affair. After reviewing their efforts to identify factors that contributed to the affair, Nick and Becky completed the worksheet shown on page 215. Later each of them used this worksheet to prepare a written narrative that expressed their best understanding of how Nick's affair had come about— a process we'll describe later in this chapter.

Nick and Becky recognized that they had gradually allowed themselves to drift apart while devoting nearly all their time and energy to

In evaluating the various factors that contributed to your relationship being at risk for an affair, be sure to include the following:

- What was going on in your relationship and with each of you before an affair was even considered

- Any experiences you and your partner had growing up in your families or with others in your life that influenced your behaviors with your partner and in regard to the affair

- What happened that actually triggered the affair

- What possibly contributed to the affair's continuing

- What has made it more difficult for you or your partner to recover

work and their children. This had interfered first with their feeling close emotionally and then with their physical intimacy. They also had given up some of their important friendships with people who had supported their relationship through difficult times in the past. Although Nick and Becky rarely had major arguments, their reluctance to address ongoing concerns in their relationship led to a steady undercurrent of tension and irritability. Their sexual relationship seemed particularly difficult to discuss. Nick and Becky also now recognized that Nick's warm and easy way of interacting with women could trigger feelings of attraction from those women that required clear boundaries, which Nick had sometimes been reluctant to set.

After ending his affair, Nick's guilt and shame had made it difficult for him to even talk with Becky about what had happened. Becky's tendency to retreat when feeling wounded and Nick's shame were barriers to working together toward recovery. Only because of their genuine caring for each other and strong desire to preserve their family were Nick and Becky able to survive Nick's affair and gradually work toward the understanding reflected in the worksheet they prepared together.

After completing this worksheet, Nick and Becky each prepared a written narrative that expressed their best understanding of how Nick's affair had come about. Both wrote their narratives in the form of a letter— something they had learned to do as a way of communicating initially about difficult issues when working through Chapter 3 and struggling with the initial impact of the affair.

Sample Worksheet Completed by Nick and Becky

	Factors having an influence before the affair	Factors having an influence during and following the affair
Negative influences and stressors (your relationship, outside factors, your partner, you)	Frequent irritability and "nitpicking" Differences in needs for spontaneity vs. predictability Low levels of physical intimacy Intrusions into relationship time from work and children Admiration and pursuit by another, combined with Nick's enduring self-doubts Nick's inattention to risks and need for boundaries	Becky's discomfort with talking about sex Nick's capacity for compartmentalizing or separating things mentally Becky's withdrawal in response to hurt or disappointment Nick's feelings of shame that blocked discussions of the affair
Positive qualities contributing to risk (your relationship, outside factors, your partner, you)	Nick's physical attractiveness and personal warmth Both partners' strong work ethic Both partners' devotion to our children	Becky's tolerance for emotional distance based on her confidence that things would eventually improve on our own Nick's reluctance to express unhappiness in our relationship
Absence of positive or protective factors that reduce the risk of an affair (your relationship, outside factors, your partner, you)	Failure to set apart time for our relationship as a couple	Both partners retreat from supportive relationships

What Does a Narrative of the Affair Look Like?

Following is Becky's initial narrative of Nick's affair—a good example of efforts to develop a picture that's both complete and balanced.

Dear Nick,

I've worked so hard to make sense of your affair. I know you've worked hard too, and I want you to know how important that has been to me. I had to know that you needed to understand this as much as I do and that you were willing to struggle through this with me. Your affair will never make complete sense to me. There were so many choice points along the way—I wish we could both go back and do things differently. I need to know that we've both learned from this—that we each understand as best we can how we ended up here. And I need to know that we're each doing everything we can to make sure that nothing like this ever happens again.

We took each other and our relationship for granted. That's hard to admit, but I believe that on some level it's true. I guess I was so certain of us that I never even imagined that our relationship could get in trouble. We each put the children first in ways that ended up not being good for us and potentially not good for them, either. And we both let work take priority, when we should have been protecting us for the sake of our family.

I know we had our differences, but none of them ever seemed that big to me. You've said that you thought I was often irritable and that you didn't think I liked you very much anymore. I think I was just always feeling under pressure to keep everything perfect and not disappoint you. Sometimes when I withdrew from you, I was just trying to give you time and space for yourself.

You've always been more comfortable with just acting on the moment, when I've preferred things to be orderly and predictable. For me, structure was how I kept our family from becoming chaotic like my own family when I was growing up. For me, routines felt safe and secure. For you, they felt controlling and restricting—and I guess I reminded you of the way your mom was with you. We've done better lately in finding a healthier balance.

You and I never really argued, and I guess that made me feel secure because we didn't have the kinds of awful fights that my parents used to have. I know we nitpicked, and I could see the pained look on your face sometimes, but you never said very much. We just went to our separate corners. We need to keep working on handling those times better. I really want you to come to me and let me know when you're feeling hurt or upset. And I'll try to do a better job of seeking you out when I see that you've pulled back.

I'll try to reach out to you when I'm feeling hurt, too. I know I tend to pull back into my shell. It's how I survive, something I learned growing up. I'll work harder at letting you know when I'm hurt or disappointed, but I need for you to be able to hear me without feeling like I'm condemning you as some terrible person. You and I both work so hard to be good people that it's hard for us to admit when we've made mistakes or fallen short. I know we've both been working on this, but I think we'll have to get even better.

Nick, I know it's hard for me to talk with you about sex. I don't understand completely why that is, but I know it's been a problem for us. With all the stresses of work and children and wanting everything at home in order, I just wasn't in the mood for sex as often as you were. And then you started to pull back from me and didn't hold me or kiss me as often, and gradually we just became more and more physically distant. Nick, I do love being touched and held by you. I don't believe you ever understood how much I missed our physical closeness, too.

When you told me about your affair, I just completely fell apart. It confirmed all my worst fears—that I couldn't compete with other women who were younger, prettier, or more successful and a part of the world where you work. I was so incredibly hurt and frightened that I couldn't even look at you because it made the pain worse. Did that make it harder for you to end it with her, when I shut down, because you were afraid of ending up completely alone?

I don't want us to stay together because of the kids. I only want us to stay together if we can devote ourselves to each other in the right ways. I don't think we can do this all on our own. Before your affair we became really isolated from our friends. I want us to start going out with other couples again, like we did before the kids were born. And I want us both to take time to renew the separate friendships that were good for us.

You know I'll never excuse your affair, and I now believe that you never will either. Nothing will ever make that affair "right." But we can try to learn from the past to make the present and our future better. I think we've been making progress, but I don't want to stop working together. There are things we each still need to work on.

I do love you, Nick. That's why this work is so important to me.

Becky

Nick's narrative was briefer. Although he understood and agreed with the contributing factors he and Becky had identified, he continued to struggle with remorse and preferred to focus on his own role. However, Becky had asked him to work with her toward the "bigger picture," and he tried to do so.

Dear Becky,

I hardly know where to begin. What I want to say most is how very sorry I am. I don't know how to express how horrible I feel every time I think about what I did. You've told me that I need to get unstuck from my guilt to focus on what needs to change, and I hope you can see now that I'm committed to doing whatever it takes to make our relationship work. I also want you to know how grateful I am that you've hung in there. I don't know if I could have been as strong as you if the situation were reversed. Your strength through this terrible ordeal is another reminder of how lucky I am to have you in my life.

Looking back, I still don't understand how I did what I did. I understand that things weren't going all that well between us at home and that we each had a lot going on in our lives. And I understand better how I've probably wrestled with feeling inadequate in one way or another for a long time. But I want you to know that—putting that all together—it still doesn't add up to what I let myself get involved in. I'll never again let myself cave in to self-pity to look for reassurance elsewhere.

Becky, maybe we both took our relationship for granted, but I probably did that the most. When you weren't there for me at times or in ways that I wanted, I felt sorry for myself. Sometimes I'd go off with my friends, and that seemed to annoy you even more. We've already talked some about how to change this. I feel good about leaving work earlier to be home for dinner and evenings with you and the kids. And I can tell the difference it's made for you, too—because you seem more relaxed and less irritated with me.

I'm sorry you thought I lost interest in you. I've always thought you were so attractive, and I loved what we did in bed together. I felt closer to you when we made love—it was the feeling between us afterward that meant the most to me. When we didn't have sex, and then we didn't have that feeling afterward, that's when I started to feel the most alone. I know I should have done a better job of explaining that, and I also should have done better at finding out what it took for you to feel closer to me. I think we've been doing a lot better in the past couple of months in finding different ways to be close together—not just sex, but other ways, too.

Becky, you're an incredible mom and you make our home a good place to live. I appreciate all you do to keep things in order and to plan special events for us. I understand better now why predictability is important to you—and how scary it must have been for you growing up when you could never predict how it was going to be at home. I think we've been getting better about this, too. I actually enjoy working with the kids after dinner to get the kitchen cleaned up so you can have time for yourself. And then going for walks or getting out of the house together for half an hour without worrying so much about chores or what the kids are doing has been a really nice change.

You've said we should go out with other couples more, and I agree. After my affair, I just couldn't bear being around other couples who seemed to get along so well because I could only think of how I betrayed you and the kids. We need to surround ourselves with other people who can support us and our relationship. It's been too easy for me to feel like the "lone ranger" out there—all alone—and I clearly got lost along the way.

Becky, I adore you. You've been the most wonderful and precious gift of my life. I will never, ever lose sight of that again, and—if you'll still have me—I promise I will do whatever it takes to keep you as the focus of my life forever.

Love, Nick

After Becky and Nick had each written their own narratives of Nick's affair, they exchanged and read them in private. They took a few days to reflect on what they had each written and then got together to discuss where they saw things similarly and where they differed. Following this discussion, Becky and Nick each revised their narratives and again exchanged and discussed them. Their revisions not only included some of the corrected understandings that had come from their previous discussion but also emphasized some of the steps they had already taken to make things better over the prior months and how those efforts had helped.

How Do I Share This Work with My Partner?

Despite your best efforts, your partner still may not be ready or willing to join you in this process. If so, consider the suggestions provided in Chapter 6 for working through this stage separately or by yourself. For example, your partner may be willing to review the worksheet of contributing factors that you've constructed (Exercise 10.1) or to read through your narrative (Exercise 10.2) and then discuss their reactions. If your partner won't participate at this level, go ahead and do this work by yourself anyway. Your partner may eventually recognize the importance of joining you in this effort. Even if your partner doesn't take part in this process, you'll have a better understanding of how the affair came about and reach better decisions about how to move forward—whether in this relationship or separately on your own—if you complete the worksheet and construct a narrative of the affair as we've described here.

EXERCISES

Complete the following exercises, first using the worksheet to summarize your understanding of the factors that contributed to the affair and then writing a narrative or story of the affair, using everything you've learned to pull together a more complete picture. Take your time. **These two exercises may be some of the most important work you'll do to recover from the affair.**

EXERCISE 10.1 Creating a Summary of Important Factors Contributing to the Affair

In this first exercise, fill in a copy of the worksheet on the next page, summarizing what you see as the important factors contributing to the affair. This worksheet can be downloaded from The Guilford Press website at *www.guilford.com/snyder2-forms*, or you can construct your own version of the same form. Look back at your responses to the exercises for Chapters 6 through 9. Try to include not only negative factors, but also positive aspects of your relationship or of you and your partner that may have been important factors. Try not to leave any portion of the worksheet entirely blank, and try to limit yourself to five or six items in any particular category.

EXERCISE 10.2 Preparing and Sharing a Narrative of the Affair

In your own words, write a narrative or story of what you see as the major factors that contributed to the development of the affair and what kept it going if it continued. Use the worksheet you just created to develop your story of how the affair came about. Remember to include any long-standing risk factors, more recent influences that may have triggered the affair or contributed to its continuing, and factors that have made it more difficult for you or your partner to recover. *In short, make sure your story of the affair has a beginning, a middle, and an end.*

If your partner hasn't been reading the book or hasn't been doing the exercises, then still write out your own story. When you've finished, ask your partner whether they'd be willing to read it and engage in a discussion with you. Even if your partner isn't willing to read or discuss your narrative, writing it will give you greater understanding, and perhaps your partner will be more willing to read it in the future.

If you and your partner are both working through these chapters, then after each of you has prepared your narrative you should exchange and discuss them, using the following steps for doing this:

Worksheet for Summarizing Factors Related to the Affair

	Factors having an influence before the affair	Factors having an influence during and following the affair
Negative influences and stressors (your relationship, outside factors, your partner, you)		
Positive qualities contributing to risk (your relationship, outside factors, your partner, you)		
Absence of positive or protective factors that reduce the risk of an affair (your relationship, outside factors, your partner, you)		

1. Exchange and read each other's narrative or story separately.

2. Discuss with your partner how you saw things similarly and differently.

3. If this discussion gives you new insights, revise your narrative, but don't feel you have to see things exactly as your partner does.

4. Exchange and discuss these changes.

5. Acknowledge any remaining differences in understanding between the two of you.

6. Focus on what you see in common and how you can use that to move forward in the future.

PART III

How Can We Move Forward?

11

How Do I Get Past the Hurt?

"I'm still having trouble getting past it," Brooke said softly. "Cody has done everything I've asked and more. For the most part, we're doing a lot better now than we were six months ago. But sometimes when I think about his affair, I still get angry and say ugly things I don't really mean, and then afterward I usually feel even worse. Most of the time, Cody just takes it or walks off without saying anything. But I know he feels beaten down when I lash out like that. Last week he asked me whether I'd ever get over it. What's that supposed to mean? I can't just forget what happened—even though I sometimes wish I could. And maybe reminding Cody of all the pain he's caused with his affair will keep him from doing something like that again. I just wish I knew what to do with the resentment I still feel and how to move on."

Even after you've worked to understand how the affair came about and addressed factors that put your relationship at risk, hurt feelings can linger. When there's little relief from the hurt and the painful feelings remain too strong or resurface too frequently, they not only get in the way of emotional closeness but eventually do even more damage to you and your relationship. Finding a way to move past the deep hurt of an affair is a crucial part of recovery.

Chronic, unresolved hurt and anger can be unhealthy, both emotionally and physically. Considerable research shows that long-lasting hurt and anger frequently lead to depression, difficulties with sleep or with appetite (eating either too little or too much), decreases in sexual desire, irritability toward friends or coworkers, high blood pressure, muscle tension, head-aches or back pain, and both emotional and physical fatigue. To counter-act these effects, some people turn to alcohol or increase their reliance on medications.

Although the research is more recent and less extensive, similar findings have emerged for persistent feelings of shame. *It's important to understand the difference between guilt and shame.* Although opinions about guilt and shame vary among mental health professionals and have evolved over the years, we believe the following viewpoint may be helpful. Specifically, we regard guilt as involving the painful feelings that result from having behaved in ways that violate one's own values. The remorse that arises from those behaviors can promote concern and empathy for those injured by the behaviors, efforts to reverse or repair their damaging impact, and healthy vigilance that reduces the likelihood of engaging in the same behaviors in the future. By contrast, shame involves a kind of self-loathing. Self-loathing rarely promotes healthy change. Instead, it can actually increase the likelihood of either unhealthy withdrawal from the situation or anger and lashing out rather than increasing concern for oth-ers; shame can feel so intolerable to the person experiencing it that they'll do almost anything to escape it.

In this chapter when we talk about getting past the hurt, we're spe-cifically addressing the kinds and depths of emotional pain that get in the way of healing and moving on in healthy ways—whether as the injured or involved partner. The goal isn't to eliminate all lingering hurt or guilt from the affair. Instead, the goal is to be certain you don't remain stuck in those feelings over the long term so they won't dominate you. The hope is that you can move past deep, intense hurt or relentless shame that consumes either partner in destructive or unhealthy ways.

The more successful you've been in working through the previous chapters, the more likely you've already made good progress in working past these kinds of hurt. But everyone is different. Some people continue to feel deep hurt that interferes with their day-to-day lives both in and outside their relationship even after working through the first two stages of recovery. Others, like Brooke, wrestle with feeling hurt and having memo-ries of the affair at least occasionally. And some remain mired in shame or deep guilt that immobilizes them, rather than drawing on deepened understanding in ways that promote awareness and change.

Deep, relentless guilt or shame can get in the way of moving forward. It can feel so overwhelming that it interferes with examining what happened or why. Learning from one's mistakes requires tolerating the discomfort that goes hand in hand with knowing you've fallen short. It requires acknowledging that we're all imperfect—and then offering compassion to our partners but also to ourselves in order to grow into a better relationship.

What does it take, then, to move past the hurt in a realistic and healthy way? In this chapter, we'll help you consider what "moving on" or "letting go" might mean and how doing so relates to beliefs you already have about forgiveness. We'll help you identify steps you or your partner can take toward moving past the hurt, as well as some of the barriers that may be making this more difficult. As you work through this chapter, however, try to remember that *feelings are usually harder to change than behaviors*. It's easier to choose how to act—and even choose how to think—than to choose how to feel. Because it's so hard to change your feelings, it's going to take time, even when you and your partner are doing everything "right." So try to be patient and encouraging to each other.

What Does It Mean to Move On?

Like Brooke, you may be struggling with questions about what it means to "move on." Does it mean never thinking about the affair again or never feeling upset about it? Does it mean no longer holding your partner or yourself accountable? When people talk about moving on, they often mean different things—in terms of what it would look like at the end or what it would take to get there. We begin with describing what moving on looks like at the end, because knowing where you want to end up is important before constructing a map that will lead you there.

Couples who move on after a deep personal injury like an affair achieve four important goals:

- They regain a balanced view of their partner, themselves, and their relationship.
- They commit to not letting their hurt, anger, or shame rule their thoughts and behaviors or dominate their lives.

■ They voluntarily stop punishing their partners or themselves for the affair but, instead, use new understandings to promote healthy change.

■ They decide whether to continue in the relationship based on a realistic assessment of both its positive and negative qualities.

Achieving a balanced view involves adopting a big-picture perspective that considers both positive and negative qualities. It requires viewing your partner and yourself not just in terms of the affair but also in light of everything else you've come to understand about yourselves and your relationship. Making a commitment not to let your hurt or anger take over your life doesn't mean never hurting again. It means working at not allowing those feelings to consume you. It requires recognizing when negative feelings about the affair resurface and then choosing to respond in ways that will be more constructive than simply lashing out. It involves redirecting your thoughts and actions toward current or future goals, rather than being overwhelmed by the past.

For some people, having the involved partner make amends can be an important part of moving on. Although nothing can undo an affair, acts of restitution or going "above and beyond" to show caring, concern, and love can sometimes serve as concrete expressions of remorse or a commitment to change. But demanding restitution—or punishing the involved partner—beyond a certain point doesn't strengthen the relationship or promote feelings of closeness. Continued vengeance may feel satisfying in the short run, but it almost always keeps you firmly stuck in the past in the long run. So, too, does relentless shame that leads you to want to escape your discomfort about the affair by withdrawing from your partner or striking back.

When people choose to stay in a relationship, moving on means committing to a process of strengthening and maintaining the relationship, even during difficult times. You haven't moved on if you stay in the relationship but with one foot out the door. Uncertainty that's allowed to drag on that way can sap the very energy necessary to make the relationship work. If, however, you choose to leave the relationship, moving on separately means no longer dwelling on the affair or your partner. It means redirecting your thoughts and behaviors toward building a new life.

Whether you stay with your partner or not, moving beyond the affair is an important part of your healing.

Moving On: Possibly Forgiving but Not Necessarily Forgetting?

Moving on, letting go, and *forgiving* are terms that people often use interchangeably. Everyone has beliefs about what it means to forgive—although often these beliefs are hard to put into words. Sometimes these beliefs come from experiences of being forgiven (or not forgiven) in the past. Maybe you have clear memories of how your parents dealt with being hurt in their own relationship or how they dealt with you when you did something that disappointed or hurt them. Or your thoughts and feelings about forgiving may be more strongly influenced by how you and your partner have dealt with hurt between you in the past. Can you remember times when you and your partner disappointed or hurt each other, but the two of you found a way to put those feelings behind you and either moved on or started fresh? Can you remember times when either one of you was unable to get past hurt feelings and what impact that had on your relationship?

People's beliefs about forgiveness are also often closely linked to religious and cultural beliefs. In some religious traditions, people are forgiven only after they've confessed to wrongdoing and expressed remorse, as well as compensated the hurt person in some way and vowed to avoid the situations that caused the hurt. In other traditions, forgiveness may be offered to someone regardless of whether the person is remorseful or takes responsibility for the hurtful behavior. From this perspective, a decision to forgive or "let go" involves giving up resentment and viewing the wrongdoer with compassion, even though the offending person may not be asking for forgiveness. What would forgiving your partner mean to you? Is forgiveness something you're willing to offer? Or if you're struggling with deep relentless guilt or shame from having an affair that blocks you from moving forward, what would it mean to forgive yourself?

It's important to understand exactly what *you* mean by forgiveness so that you know what you can live with and in what ways you truly want to move on. Does forgiving mean pardoning to you? Pardoning someone for an offense generally releases that person from further punishment or restitution—without necessarily having any implications for how you feel about the person. For most people forgiving goes beyond pardoning: When you forgive someone, you also experience some "softening of the heart" toward that person. To reconcile with someone, in contrast, means to restore a healed relationship—not just staying or moving back in together, but joining with one another on a deeper secure level. Although it's probably impossible to reconcile in that way without first forgiving, people can forgive without reconciling. For example, you could say to someone, "I no longer want to punish you. I understand what led you to do what you did. I can see your remorse, and I'm sorry for your own suffering. However, I don't believe this relationship can be a healthy one for me, and I need to end it."

There's no doubt that forgiveness is a profound concept, so it's no wonder that it's often misunderstood or viewed in ways that are not helpful. *Some common beliefs about forgiveness can actually interfere with moving on—for example*:

- I need to forgive someone who apologizes, whether I want to or not.
- Forgiving someone means excusing what they did or saying that what happened is okay.
- Forgiving someone for hurtful or wrong actions requires compromising my own values regarding what's right.
- Some behaviors (for example, affairs or violence) shouldn't be forgiven.
- Forgiveness can't occur until compensation or restitution has been made.
- To forgive someone means no longer thinking about what that person did.
- Forgiving someone means no longer feeling hurt or angry about what happened.
- Forgiving someone means leaving myself open to being hurt again.
- If I forgive someone, I need to stay in a relationship with that person.

Have you held beliefs similar to any of these? Which ones stand out for you? Would you add any? Try looking at these beliefs in light of what we've discussed so far. How might any of these beliefs be helpful to you in moving past your own hurt feelings—and how might they get in the way? Let us make our own views on the meaning of forgiveness clear:

- *Forgiving someone—whether your partner or yourself—**doesn't** mean approving of what was done.* No matter how understanding you may be about what contributed to the affair, you're unlikely ever to believe that it was the right choice or a good one.

- *Similarly, forgiving someone **isn't** the same as excusing or justifying what was done.* You and your partner may have worked hard to understand how the affair came about or what factors put your relationship at risk. But contributing factors aren't excuses, just as explanations aren't justifications.

- *Finally, forgiving someone **doesn't** mean forgetting about the offense or no longer hurting from it.* You and your partner will continue to have times when you think about the affair, and those times may be accompanied by feelings of hurt, resentment, guilt, anxiety, or sadness. But moving on means working to minimize those thoughts and feelings by focusing on opportunities for pursuing a happy and productive life now and in the future. *By itself, the passage of time helps but rarely heals deep emotional wounds.* Moving on, letting go, and forgiving all require commitment to a process that will help you reach this goal and actively taking steps to move forward.

What Are the Steps to Moving On?

There's no single sequence of events or universal time line that works well for everyone. The specific steps may vary, depending on the factors contributing to the affair, your beliefs about forgiveness, your partner's behaviors, and consequences of the affair for you or for others—such as your children. The steps we'll describe over the next few pages represent a process that fits for many people. Not all of these steps may be relevant or essential for your own moving on, and the order of these steps may be different for you. Use the following discussion and Exercise 11.1 to think about what actions seem important to *you* for moving on. Which of these have you and your partner already achieved? Which ones still lie before you—and how could you help to bring these about?

As you consider each of the steps described below, reflect on what you've learned and worked on in previous chapters. Although the involved partner owns sole responsibility for the decision to have an affair, each of you may have identified ways you contributed to your relationship becoming vulnerable. What have you learned about your own roles in your relationship prior to the affair that potentially contributed to risk? Have you acknowledged this to your partner? Knowing what you know now, what changes have you committed yourself to, and how successfully have you implemented these?

Recognition

Step 1 involves developing a clear understanding of what happened and its consequences. Think back to the material in Chapter 3 about discussing your feelings about the affair. Did you and your partner exchange letters as suggested in the exercises for that chapter? If not, were you able to have a thorough and helpful discussion about the impact of the affair? If you didn't complete the exercises for that chapter or if important aspects of understanding the impact of the affair still seem not to be recognized or understood, reread that chapter or ask your partner to read and discuss the chapter with you.

Responsibility

Affairs don't "just happen." They involve a decision—either explicit or implicit—to cross the line and engage in a behavior that almost always has been defined or understood ahead of time by the couple as not acceptable. Couples can get stuck in the recovery process, and injured partners can find it particularly difficult to move past their hurt if the involved partner persists in declaring, "I never meant to hurt you." Although usually not intended as such, this statement can convey a continued failure to take responsibility for avoiding or actively resisting an affair. Injured partners frequently can't move on until the person who had the affair takes responsibility for their choices throughout the affair and makes a genuine effort to understand why they made those choices. Similarly, depending on what you learned in Part II of the book, the involved partner may find it difficult to feel hopeful if the injured partner doesn't consider their own contributions to the relationship becoming at risk.

Remorse

What would it mean if someone hurt you, acknowledged what they had done, recognized the painful impact, and took responsibility for their actions—but then had no feelings of remorse for what they did? That person would seem insensitive and uncaring, if not spiteful or even cruel. Declaring and showing remorse are ways of saying and truly experiencing, "It hurts me to know that I've put you through such pain. Your distress is now my distress—even more so because I'm the one who caused you to hurt." Remorse goes beyond accepting responsibility for hurting someone. To have remorse is to feel deep sadness, mourning, or even pain from the hurt you've brought to another person. Remorse indicates that your partner's pain *matters* to you. Remorse can also involve a deep regret about acting outside of your own value system; as an involved partner, not only did you let down your partner, you may have let down yourself as well.

Restitution

When you do something wrong and hurt someone you love, often there's a desire to do something good to make up for the wrong or to make the bad feelings go away; these are acts of restitution. Although nothing can undo an affair, there are many things that someone can do to concretely demonstrate feelings of remorse and perhaps reduce the distress of their partner. For example, in responding to Brooke's deep hurt from his affair, Cody told her:

> "I know that I can never make up for the terrible pain that I've caused you, and I will always feel horrible about that. But I will try as best I can to show you my commitment by being less selfish and treating you more kindly. I know that it used to disappoint you that I spent much of my free time with my friends instead of with you, and I'm committed to changing that. I used to ignore your needs for a break from the kids and time with your own friends, and I'm determined to make sure you have at least one

evening each week to spend with your friends. I can never undo what I did, but I can promise to do a better job of loving you."

It's important to distinguish between restitution and revenge. Restitution is a partner's attempt to balance the scales by engaging in important *positive* actions. By contrast, in revenge an injured person tries to "even things up" by retaliating with *negative* behaviors. Revenge may feel satisfying in the short run, but it rarely promotes healing in the long run; instead, it just maintains or intensifies the negative feelings or behaviors.

As an injured partner, you need to examine the extent to which making amends is important for you to move forward. As an involved partner, it's important to recognize that moving on past the trauma of your affair will probably occur sooner or more fully when you work at caring for your partner's distress and nurturing your relationship. This is important to do even if the injured partner doesn't seem to acknowledge these efforts or doesn't respond in a positive way. You may have to persist at efforts to make restitution before things improve.

Reform

It's difficult to move beyond deep hurt unless you're assured that the person who caused the harm has committed not to behave in the same way again. The involved partner needs to commit to making necessary changes to reduce the likelihood that this will happen again.

Efforts toward reform include three steps:

1. Pledging never to hurt one's partner in the same way again
2. Addressing conditions that contributed to the affair
3. Acting differently when confronted with similar situations in the future

It's not realistic for partners to promise never to hurt one another at any level or in any form. But it *is* realistic to commit to avoiding certain hurtful behaviors—such as keeping secrets or engaging in inappropriate sexual or emotionally intimate relationships with others outside of agreed-upon boundaries. Pursuing reform involves addressing and minimizing the contributing factors that you and your partner have identified that previously placed your relationship at risk for an affair. That includes not only addressing relationship issues such as levels of conflict or intimacy, but also continuing to work on individual issues (such as concerns about physical attractiveness or sexual adequacy) that contributed to having an affair. Promising to act differently is important to reform, but what's essential is actually *behaving* differently when temptations or opportunities for affairs arise. Evidence of reform helps to reestablish feelings of safety and trust that promote letting go of past hurt and moving on.

Release

Release comes closest to what we think of as the core of forgiveness. Release involves freeing both yourself and your partner from further punishment and from being dominated by deep hurt, anger, guilt, or shame that lingers after the affair. Release doesn't mean approval; it doesn't mean forgetting or no longer hurting. Rather, committing to release involves an explicit decision to work toward a process of moving on.

> Mario and Alba had worked together for almost a year to rebuild their relationship following Alba's affair. But Mario continued to wrestle with memories of Alba's affair and the hurt and resentment toward Alba that these memories stirred up. "I can't just wipe the slate clean," he shared with his closest friend. "That seems like forgetting it ever happened, and I'm afraid that we could slip back into our old ways that weren't working."
>
> Alba's remorse was evident to Mario, as were the many ways she had worked to improve their relationship. Mario wrestled with his attitudes about forgiveness, and a month later he declared to his friend, "I think I've come to a decision about how to do this better. I can't fully erase what she's done, but I can set it aside and start fresh. Setting it aside means we're removing it from being at the center of our lives and, instead, making our new relationship our focus."

Reconciliation

Recovery from an affair doesn't necessarily mean reconciling or staying in your relationship. In the next chapter, we'll help you draw on everything you've learned and worked on to reach a well-informed decision about how to move forward—either in this relationship or separately.

But for some couples who work through the recovery process together—particularly those who follow a process similar to the one we've outlined in this book—reconciliation results from going through the previous steps we've described for moving on.

> When Jeremy returned from an assignment overseas, Lauren sensed that something was different. After first denying that anything was wrong, Jeremy confessed that he had been sexually intimate on two occasions with another woman while away. He had no wish to continue his relationship with the other person on any level but described feeling deeply confused about his feelings for Lauren. Jeremy felt tremendous remorse for his affair but also wondered whether he could truly still love Lauren, given what he had done. His affair didn't make sense to either of them.
>
> Jeremy and Lauren spent several months examining the emotional distance that had grown between them in recent years. Although clear from the beginning that they wanted to save their relationship, it was eight months before Lauren was able to move beyond her deep hurt and Jeremy beyond his own equally deep guilt. They decided to go away for a weekend to one of their favorite places in the mountains, where they renewed their vows of commitment to one another. The ritual that Jeremy and Lauren created symbolized their reconciliation and the promise of their new beginning.

What Are the Barriers to Moving On?

Understanding the steps to moving on past deep relationship hurt can be useful in understanding where you are in the process of recovering from the affair. However, it's also important to understand some of the barriers that can make this process more difficult.

Continued Hurtful Actions (or Inactions) of Your Partner

You may find it difficult to move on if your partner continues to behave in ways that contribute to your feeling hurt or insecure in the relationship. Your partner may continue to do things that used to be okay but that you now find difficult to accept because of their association with the affair.

No matter how innocent they may be, separate evenings out with friends, trips out of town, or late nights at work can easily trigger memories and feelings related to the affair. And, of course, any continued contact with the outside person inevitably stirs up continued apprehension, hurt, or resentment about the affair. The bottom line is this: *What once may have been entirely innocent and "safe" behaviors may no longer be acceptable or may interfere with moving on because of their association with the deeply painful affair.*

Both you and your partner need to examine carefully any potential pitfalls along these lines so you can eliminate as many of them as possible. Build in temporary safety measures that help to reduce anxieties and hurt feelings from the affair—such as regularly checking in by phone when separated, arranging for other trusted workers to be present when working late, or avoiding situations that unnecessarily stir up thoughts and feelings related to the affair.

Ultimately, you and your partner will need to collaborate in defining new arrangements that can be tolerated by both of you. These new limits or requirements won't work for your relationship if they're so harsh or punitive as to create resentment or push your partner away. But they may need to be more restrictive than before the affair—at least for a while—to help you in moving past the hurt and until trust can be rebuilt.

Beliefs about Forgiveness

Read again through the list of common beliefs about forgiveness on page 232 and ask yourself whether any of these apply to you and whether they're making it more difficult for you to move on. For example, do you worry that if you let go of your hurt and became emotionally close to your partner, you might leave yourself open to being hurt by another affair? Are you concerned that committing to moving on would imply forgetting the affair or minimizing the damage it caused? Consider whether any of these beliefs are getting in the way of moving on and how a different perspective might work better for you. For example, if the idea of "wiping the slate clean" doesn't work for you, could you consider keeping that slate but setting it aside and then working with your partner toward writing a new one?

Fear of Being Hurt Again

The fear of another affair often provokes a constant state of vigilance—mentally rehearsing what happened in the past and scanning your environment to look for evidence of it happening again. Constantly reliving the trauma of the affair keeps alive not just the memories but also the deep hurt feelings. We don't encourage you to stay in a relationship dominated by betrayals and mistrust. But "trust"—by definition—is different from "certainty." *Trust requires acting without knowing for sure what will happen.* For example, if you observe that the sun rises each morning and falls at night, you probably aren't constantly looking out your window to check if it's still in the sky. *That* is trust. You trust that the sun will be there, even though you can't really do anything to guarantee that it will.

If you've followed the process outlined in this book, you and your partner have already done a lot to reduce the likelihood that an affair will happen again. Yet still, the future will always be at least a little uncertain. If you decide to stay in your relationship, you'll have to choose to *trust* in your partner above and beyond the work you've done thus far. You'll need to decide whether, based on everything you know about your partner and your relationship, you're willing to work toward rebuilding trust. If so, understand that doing so inevitably involves accepting some degree of risk of being hurt again—no matter how small. Holding on to your hurt or always checking up on your partner to make sure they aren't having another affair won't eliminate that risk, and continuing to pull away from or lash out at your partner could eventually increase that risk.

Reluctance to Give Up Status as the Injured Party

Being the injured person provides an opportunity to claim the moral high ground by having been wronged. We've seen injured partners who have used their status as the offended person to maintain leverage in their relationship by demanding continued apologies, concessions, or reparations. We've also known injured partners who have used their hurt feelings from the affair as a reason for continuing to lash out and punish the involved partner long after the affair has ended. There's a fine line between requiring reform or restitution as a basis for moving on past hurt feelings and using hurt feelings as a way of maintaining influence or inflicting further hurt in a relationship. If you're having difficulty letting go, consider whether any part of your difficulty relates to advantages in the relationship you might need to give up by deciding to forgive or move on.

Potential Barriers for Involved Partners

Involved partners can also struggle with issues of forgiveness, particularly forgiving themselves for an affair. For example, if you're the involved partner, you may fear that forgiving yourself would make it easier to forget what happened and let down your guard against hurting your partner again. You may be reluctant to seek your partner's forgiveness because you believe doing so would imply seeking pardon or acceptance for what you did. Or you may believe that you need to continue suffering at least as long as your partner suffers.

In the short run, appropriate levels of guilt can promote changes in your own behavior that are difficult to make. But excessive guilt or shame tends to immobilize people and undermine constructive change. Not just for your own sake, but for your partner's and your relationship's sake, examine whether deep guilt, shame, or anger toward yourself is interfering with restoring a joyful and secure relationship. Consider factors that could be keeping you stuck—including beliefs about forgiveness or advantages you may be reluctant to give up by holding on to your deep guilt or shame (for example, lessening your partner's wish to punish you or seek further restitution). Consider also the risks of not forgiving yourself and moving on. How could moving past relentless shame be helpful not only to you but also to your relationship?

Are Some Affairs Harder to Heal from than Others?

Healing from an affair is hard. It's complicated and often not straightforward. However, there are numerous factors sometimes related to an affair that can make recovery even more difficult. One way of thinking about these complicating factors is to consider them according to whether they relate primarily to the past, present, or future.

Making Sense of the Past

An important part of healing from an affair is making sense of what's already happened. The "bigger" the affair and betrayal, the harder it's likely to be to make sense of it and move forward. Affairs can feel "bigger" than usual for various reasons. For example, the length of the affair can impact recovery. When you first learned of your partner's affair, you may have felt like you'd been living a fantasy—that your life wasn't what you had thought it was. So the longer the affair lasted, the more your life might feel like one big illusion. No affair that violates your boundaries is okay, but a one-night stand under unusual circumstances might be less difficult to recover from than learning that your partner's been continuing a close, intimate relationship with someone else for months or years, living a kind of dual life that you didn't know about. How do you make sense of an entire reality you didn't even know existed?

Similar to a long-term affair, the timing of when you learn about the affair might also impact how you recover. For example, we've worked with couples in which a partner learns about an affair that happened years or decades earlier in the couple's relationship. In some ways, this might seem less painful because it's in the distant past. However, for some injured partners it becomes even harder to recover because they now question the last 20 or 30 years of their relationship—struggling with what's been real and what's been rooted in deception.

An affair also can feel "bigger" and be more difficult to heal from depending on who the outside person was. Did the affair involve a "double" betrayal in some sense? For example, was the outside person someone that you knew and perhaps trusted—a friend, colleague, or even a family member? Such double betrayals almost always make healing from an affair more difficult. Or did someone close to you know about the affair but not tell you, continuing to interact with you as if nothing was happening? Feelings of betrayal multiply, and recovery becomes more difficult, when other people in your life were involved in the infidelity either directly or indirectly, leading you to feel that you can't know whom to trust or whether any boundaries are truly secure.

A similar complicating factor arises if the affair was with someone who was in a trusted position with you or your partner, or with the two of you as a couple. There are various circumstances when we may place certain people in unique positions of trust so that we can open up to them in vulnerable ways we wouldn't ordinarily do with others. For example, we take off our clothes in front of medical personnel, or we might reveal our innermost thoughts and feelings to a therapist, counselor, or religious leader. This is always done with the understanding that the person in that trusted position won't use our vulnerability, what they learn about us, or their power to harm us. If you've experienced such a violation from someone you've held in trust, then not only has your partner betrayed you but so too have important institutions in your life and the people representing those institutions. Violations of this sort invariably make healing from an affair more difficult.

Experiencing the Present

Even if you've done a good job of making sense of the past, what happened doesn't just go away—it's still a part of your present life. For example, there will be times or situations that trigger strong feelings related to the affair—perhaps the anniversary of when you found out about the affair or when driving by some location that reminds you of the outside person. However, the consequences of some affairs may increase the frequency or depth of those feelings in ongoing, unavoidable ways. For example, if a child was born as a result of the affair, that outcome may continue to trigger painful memories and harsh interactions with your partner or child in unintended ways that might confuse you both. Or if your partner contracted a sexually transmitted infection and passed it on to you, you may now experience physical as well as emotional distress from the affair in ways that repeatedly trigger painful reminders. Even less dramatic but enduring consequences—for example, disruptions to important social, faith-based, or family relationships, or financial strains from changes at work resulting from the affair—may serve as triggers that continue to bring the whole thing back to you at unexpected times in ways that make it more difficult to heal and move on.

Predicting the Future

How you think about your future will also impact your ability to move forward. Healing and moving forward with your partner require a sense of safety and predictability to give you confidence that you won't be hurt again in similar ways; therefore, any aspects of the affair that increase the risk of similar events in the future will likely cause you to be more cautious and make recovery more difficult. For example, if your partner has had multiple affairs in the past even after the two of you worked to address them as a couple, then reconciling and moving forward with your partner might be a higher risk. Similarly, if you've been hurt by an ex-partner's affair or have had other people in your life betray you in some way, then recovery from this most recent affair might be more difficult for you because your experiences over time may have built a reservoir of mistrust. If that's the case for you, try to separate your partner's actions from the betrayal of others so you can deal with your current situation for what it is.

Likewise, how your partner makes sense of the affair could detract from their commitment to making important changes. If your partner doesn't take responsibility for their role in the affair or makes statements such as "I was drunk and didn't know what I was doing," "It wasn't my fault; the other person was pursuing me," or "It was your best friend; of course I trusted him," then moving forward will likely be more difficult for you, even if there's some kernel of truth in what your partner is saying. A partner's failure to own responsibility for their own behaviors and to make necessary, difficult changes invariably makes it difficult to trust the future.

Finally, if your partner remains in high-risk situations for boundary violations or inappropriate behaviors with others, recovery will likely be more difficult—even if your partner is motivated to change. For example, if future circumstances call for your partner to continue interactions with the outside person or be placed in situations similar to that in which the infidelity occurred previously, then the risk goes up and your feelings of safety go down. So if circumstances could place your partner in high-risk situations in the future, it's important that you both acknowledge this and work together toward minimizing or safeguarding those situations as best as possible.

Healing from Complicated Affairs

You can't undo the past, but you can likely take steps to deal with these more complicating aspects of affairs to achieve your own goals for recovery. For example, if the affair lasted for years and you now have to figure out what was real and what was fantasy in your relationship, then both you and your partner need to pursue important but difficult conversations about what that period of life was like for both of you. *It's hard to move on when you don't know what you're moving on from.* Or if the affair included other important people in your life either as the outside person or others who knew about the affair but didn't tell you, then you and your partner will need to decide whether to confront those persons or possibly the institutions they represent, recognizing potential risks or negative consequences of those confrontations. For example, if the affair was with a coworker or a family member, do you risk your broader family knowing or people in the workplace spreading the word in damaging ways? If the outside person was part of an agency or institution that you trusted, do you notify the institution or initiate a formal complaint that could risk the person's licensure or job? You may well decide that this is appropriate and important to pursue, but make sure you understand the possible implications of such a process for either you or your partner so that you can reach an informed decision together. In some instances, it might be valuable to seek confidential input from others with relevant experience or expertise.

In dealing with ongoing emotional triggers, there's a complicated balancing act you need to navigate. On the one hand, you should avoid engaging unnecessarily in situations likely to trigger painful reactions—for example, socializing with the outside person, looking at the outside person's social media page, or watching movies involving infidelity during a date night. On the other hand, if you're trying to avoid or deny what happened or overly restricting your world to avoid emotional triggers, you might be allowing the past to control your present and future in unhealthy ways. The optimal balance of minimizing versus tolerating triggers may vary over time. For example, immediately after learning about your partner's affair, you may need to take care of yourself by avoiding certain situations likely to intensify painful emotions. But as you work through the recovery process we've described and those emotions hopefully decrease, it might be important to expand your world and reduce your avoidance—always reevaluating when, where, and how to engage emotional triggers in ways that allow you to live the fullest life possible.

In terms of the future, you should evaluate the likelihood that future affairs might occur, in line with what we've discussed throughout this book. *Whereas the past can be a good predictor of the future, neither your partner nor you are destined to repeat the past.* Your goal is to evaluate whether there are additional complicating factors or changes that you and your partner are willing to make so that the past doesn't repeat itself. In the following pages we discuss what might help if you're feeling stuck, regardless of how complicated the affair might have been.

How Do I Get Unstuck?

If you're still having difficulty moving beyond intense hurt, anger, or shame left over from the affair, pursue the additional steps described below.

Evaluate the Risks and Benefits of Moving On

The primary risk of moving on is opening oneself to being hurt again. Another barrier can be a reluctance to give up extra influence or clout afforded to an injured party. However, continued domination of a relationship through righteous hurt or anger eventually destroys any opportunity to rebuild a healthy relationship. Fostering feelings of deep guilt or shame in your partner by holding on to your own hurt or anger eventually changes guilt into resentment. In contrast, letting go of past hurt often serves as a powerful gift that not only promotes better emotional and physical health in both of you but frequently inspires your partner to work harder on behalf of the relationship and give more in return.

Make a Decision to Forgive or Move On

In his book *Forgiveness Is a Choice,* Robert Enright emphasizes that letting go of one's hurt and forgiving the wrongdoer are choices that one is free to either accept or reject. The decision to forgive doesn't mean that you've completed the process, but rather that you've made "a good beginning" in committing to the process. Making a decision to move past your hurt, anger, or shame requires you to have a vision of how you want to be emotionally, relationally, and perhaps spiritually—and commit to a process that has greater potential to get you there. Exercise 11.2 can help you in this process.

From time to time, you're still likely to have negative thoughts and feelings related to the affair even after reaching a decision to forgive or move on. If you find yourself in this situation to a degree that disrupts your efforts to move forward, the following guidelines may help.

■ *Find more constructive ways of venting your feelings.* Although sometimes it may be important to share your hurt feelings with your partner (for example, explaining that you need some time by yourself before you can resume interacting in a warm or intimate way), it's also important that you have ways of expressing your feelings separately from your partner. Alternative ways of venting your feelings include keeping a journal or sharing your feelings with a trusted friend, keeping in mind the guidelines for this included in Chapter 4.

■ *Work toward developing more effective techniques for managing your feelings when they threaten to escalate out of control.* Be sure to recognize when your feelings may be getting out of control—such as when you're having particularly "hot thoughts," having muscle tightness or other physical signs of tension, speaking in a harsh or angry manner, slamming doors, or experiencing other cues of escalating anger that you've learned to recognize. Use some of the techniques for managing intense feelings outlined in Chapter 3—using meditation or relaxation, going for a walk, engaging in moderate exercise, or taking a time-out until your feelings are under better control.

■ *Develop more effective techniques for disrupting negative thoughts that interfere with more positive feelings or constructive behaviors.* Recognizing repetitive negative thoughts and simply telling yourself to "stop" can sometimes be helpful, as can limiting your time for having such thoughts to a particular time of day or set period (for example, for 15 minutes but not longer). Redirecting your thoughts to a different topic or distracting yourself by engaging in a different activity can also help. This isn't denial—but about exercising more control over whether you dwell on negative thoughts in ways that aren't helpful.

Another way of disrupting negative thoughts is to think about things from a different, more positive perspective. For example, rather than focusing on painful memories of the affair, remind yourself that the memories aren't nearly as frequent or devastating as they once were. Or focus on the progress you and your partner have already made toward rebuilding a joyful and secure relationship.

    ■ *Work toward developing compassion for your partner.* Continue to work at understanding how your partner came to act in a hurtful way and recognize your partner's own distress and human shortcomings. Compassion comes from caring for your partner and wishing an end to your partner's own pain—whether you're the injured or involved partner.

    ■ *Draw on spiritual or similar resources that help to provide meaning in letting go and strengthen your efforts toward this goal.* If continued anger, guilt, or shame interferes with your efforts to move on for the sake of your partner or your relationship, you can still work toward forgiveness based on personal or spiritual values. Drawing on such values can help you work toward letting go of the past even when you don't feel like doing so.

    ■ *Express your desire to forgive or move on and describe steps you're willing to take toward this process.* Making an explicit declaration to your partner about your commitment to moving on can promote greater understanding and patience from your partner when you experience setbacks in letting go and may help your partner with letting go of hurt or resentment from the past as well. It's important that you both understand that your commitment to moving on implies a process that is still unfolding, not an end state that has already been achieved. It doesn't mean you won't continue to remember or hurt from the affair. It means you no longer allow hurt, anger, guilt, or shame to rule your life and you voluntarily commit to no longer punishing your partner or yourself for the affair or demanding further restitution.

    ■ *Consider getting outside professional help for managing difficult feelings or reaching challenging decisions.* Review guidelines we offered for seeking professional help in Chapter 5. Remember that getting outside help isn't weak or self-indulgent; it's about becoming healthy again for yourself and for the sake of those you care about and who care about you.

    Whether you're the injured or involved partner, work through the following exercises. These can help you examine where you are currently in the process of moving on and then reach and implement a decision to let go of deep hurt, anger, or shame that continues to damage you or your relationship.

EXERCISES

EXERCISE 11.1 Examining Your Progress toward Moving On

Make two lists. First, list steps you and your partner have already accomplished in moving on or making things better. For example, you might recognize that the involved partner has taken full responsibility for the affair and no longer engages in flirtatious or other inappropriate behaviors with others. Or perhaps you realize that earlier the injured partner often sought to hurt the involved partner with painful reminders of the affair but now tries to avoid doing this.

Second, list the steps you still need to take to move forward and clarify the barriers that are making these difficult or holding you back. For example, the injured partner might realize a need to begin showing greater trust in the involved partner—such as deciding on reasonable limits for the involved partner's behavior and then giving them a chance to demonstrate their trustworthiness. Or perhaps you or your partner have slipped into old patterns that previously put your relationship at risk— for example, devoting too many hours to work or other activities outside the home and neglecting your relationship when together. If you or your partner recognize this as a barrier to moving on, you need to work toward establishing healthier limits on outside involvements and better ways of connecting with each other.

EXERCISE 11.2 Reaching a Decision to Let Go of the Deep Hurt, Anger, or Shame

First, list the potential risks and benefits of letting go of your feelings of hurt, anger, or shame. Then list the benefits and risks of not letting go.

An example from the injured partner:

"I'm afraid that if I let go of my anger, my partner will go back to her old ways. But I also know that, in the long run, a strong relationship needs to be based on love, not anger or fear."

An example from the involved partner:

"I've hurt my partner so badly, I can't imagine not having this deep guilt and shame. But I also know I've committed to doing whatever it takes to heal from the affair, and punishing myself every day will eventually beat me down and not help my partner or our relationship."

Second, consider strategies you can implement if you continue to feel stuck despite your decision to move on. Negative feelings often continue long term because they're related to how you think about things.

An example from the injured partner:

"I know that continuing to dwell on each time you lied to me just keeps my anger alive. I want to remind myself of efforts you've made to improve our relationship and demonstrate your commitment to rebuilding trust."

An example from the involved partner:

"I never want to forget what I did or the harm I caused you and our relationship. But I want to use that to remind myself every day about what I need to do better to strengthen and protect what we have now and in the future, not to beat myself up."

12

Can This Relationship Be Saved?

Kyle and Mariana had been struggling to recover from Mariana's affair for six months, but Kyle continued to wrestle with the pain of her betrayal. The couple's work toward recovery had begun as a last-ditch effort to determine whether their relationship could be saved. Over the past six months, they had made progress in talking about their feelings and making better decisions about how to spend their time together at home. It had taken a while before Kyle started to warm up again, but Mariana had been patient. Eventually Kyle no longer had the same deep bitterness toward Mariana he had felt initially, and at times things between them seemed back to normal.

Still, some of the hurtful consequences of Mariana's affair continued. For Kyle, something in their relationship seemed lost forever. He could no longer view Mariana in the same way. He and Mariana had restored a decent friendship, but the laughter and delight they had once enjoyed with each other hadn't returned. Kyle didn't want to move on separately without Mariana, but he also didn't want to spend the rest of his life in a relationship that lacked real intimacy or passion. Would those feelings of trust ever come back? How long would it take? If they never came back, would he be able to accept that but stay with Mariana? Or would he and Mariana be better off ending their relationship as friends and moving on separately?

Some couples, like Kyle and Mariana, work hard to understand the affair and restore a caring relationship but continue to struggle to recapture feelings of trust, intimacy, or joy with each other. Even after getting beyond the intense anger related to the affair, deciding whether to move on together or separately can be difficult. In this chapter we'll help you arrive at an explicit decision about how to move forward—either by staying with your partner and recommitting to your relationship or by moving on separately. You may already have decided how to move forward. If so, we still encourage you to read this chapter and work through the exercises. Doing so may help you form clearer reasons for your decision or help you discuss this decision with your partner more effectively. Examining the issues considered here may also help you anticipate work that you or your partner may still need to pursue either to help your relationship succeed or to lead fulfilling lives separately.

What Are My Choices?

Following an affair, some people know immediately that they want to restore their relationship, while others choose at the outset to move on separately. Most people, however—particularly injured partners—have mixed feelings. Many would like to rebuild their relationship but feel too frightened, hurt, or angry to know if this is possible. Others lean toward separation but don't want to give up on their relationship without first making every possible effort to reconcile. Ultimately, the paths for moving forward fall into four types:

1. **Moving on together in a healthy way.** Some couples commit to rebuilding their relationship and do the work needed to make this happen. Both partners manage their own feelings of hurt, anger, or shame in ways that permit positive steps toward restoring trust and intimacy. The affair isn't forgotten, but it serves as a reminder of the need to continually nurture and strengthen their relationship and deal with stresses or conflicts as they arise.

2. **Moving on together in an unhealthy way.** Other couples may stay together following a partner's affair but do so poorly. They continue to interact in hurtful ways—damaging each other's relationships with their children or with others, having frequent or intense arguments, or failing to reestablish a positive relationship. If not actively hurtful in their

exchanges, partners remain isolated in emotional retreat. Persistent deep feelings of hurt, anger, or mistrust block necessary steps toward restoring a constructive and intimate relationship.

3. **Moving on separately in a healthy way.** Partners may also decide to end their relationship in a way that is least hurtful to themselves and to others they love, including their children and extended families. They work hard not to inflict further damage on each other either during or following the process of separation. If they have children, they work together to protect the emotional and physical well-being of those children. They each use what they've learned from the affair to establish happy and productive lives, either alone or in a healthy relationship with someone new.

4. **Moving on separately in an unhealthy way.** Other partners end their relationship but continue to interact in hurtful ways. Similar to those who stay together in unhealthy ways, they damage each other's relationships with their children, respective families, or friends and colleagues. Or they cut off all further contact but continue to relive previous conflicts or trauma related to the affair in their minds. Their lingering bitterness or wounded feelings often interfere with forming healthy new intimate relationships and can have a lasting negative impact on their children's intimate relationships as well.

Of course, no one actively seeks the unhealthy options. But some people end up there by default—by failing to choose and commit to the healthier alternatives. Moving on in a healthy way, either together or separately, requires you to carefully evaluate the resources and potential risks that you each bring to your relationship, decide to stay together or not, and then commit to implementing that decision as constructively as possible.

How Do I Decide?

It's not uncommon for people to have mixed feelings about their relationship, particularly when they've experienced frequent or intense arguing or gone through long periods of loneliness or emotional withdrawal. After an affair, mixed feelings are more often the norm than the exception. It may be that no decision you reach about your relationship will feel absolutely certain to you. However, it's important to struggle through your mixed feelings and try to reach a decision to move forward in one direction or the other. Evaluating what you've learned about your partner, your relationship, and yourself is vital to reaching the right decision.

Evaluating Your Partner

Think back to aspects of your partner that you considered in working through prior chapters. If you're the injured person, what did you conclude about your partner's character? Was your partner's affair an isolated event or, instead, part of a long series of betrayals or self-centered actions? Alternatively, did the affair stem in part from positive aspects of your partner that played out in an unhealthy way—including emotional sensitivity or needs for connection? Did your partner's affair occur during a time of serious relationship problems?

Has your partner accepted responsibility for the affair and expressed genuine remorse? Has your partner demonstrated the ability to make difficult changes in the past—including changes unrelated to your relationship? Consider whether your partner has implemented important changes since the affair—for example, no longer placing him- or herself in situations that encouraged inappropriate behaviors with others. Have your partner's interactions with the outside affair person been eliminated entirely or restricted to those absolutely essential because of a shared work setting?

If you're the involved partner struggling with a decision about how to move forward, evaluating factors related to the injured partner is equally important. For example, has your partner been willing to examine their own contributions to your relationship that may have placed it at greater risk for an affair? Has your partner shown progress in working past deep hurt or anger from your affair? Keep in mind that injured partners typically require a much longer time to recover from an affair than involved partners. So it may be important to remain patient for now and to focus on how to move forward within your relationship as best you can until you're fairly certain that either (1) your injured partner won't be able to restore a close, joyful relationship with you regardless of time and efforts or (2) regardless of your partner's decision and ability to recover, you want to end the relationship and move on separately.

Evaluating Your Relationship

Review the factors in your relationship you identified previously that potentially increased its vulnerability to an affair. To what extent have you and your partner addressed these concerns? For example, if you previously had frequent or intense conflicts before the affair, have you developed more effective strategies for managing your differences and reaching decisions together? If your relationship became vulnerable partly because of feeling disconnected from each other, have you found more effective ways to promote emotional or physical intimacy?

Even if your relationship prior to the affair was mostly satisfying for you both, the trauma of the affair almost certainly caused significant distress and may have produced lingering negative effects. If the affair created new problems in your relationship—for example, conflicts regarding interactions with family or friends—consider whether you've been able to work together to resolve them or are headed in that direction. Have you found ways to laugh together or do some of the things you used to enjoy as a couple? Do you and your partner share a common vision of how you'd like to move forward as a couple?

In addition, think about your relationship from the larger perspective. Why did you and your partner decide to become a couple, and how has your relationship helped you grow? Consider what you've done best together and what challenges you've overcome. Can you recover enough of what previously was good in your relationship?

Evaluating Yourself

As the injured partner, you need ways to manage your feelings so that you don't continue to lash out destructively at your partner or become overwhelmed with feelings of despair. You also need to examine aspects of yourself that may have contributed to your relationship's becoming vulnerable to an affair. For example, if difficulties in expressing feelings effectively contributed to intense arguments or emotional distance between the two of you, you need more constructive ways of discussing those feelings. Regardless of your decision to stay in this relationship or not, it's important that you find ways to move past your deep hurt to focus on the life ahead of you. Finally, if you decide to stay in this relationship, it will be important to rediscover or promote new ways of pursuing joy and intimacy with your partner. Are you willing to take gradual, appropriate risks in restoring trust in your partner and intimacy in your relationship?

If you're the involved partner, you have challenges of your own to address in deciding how to move forward. Have you honestly examined aspects of yourself that led to your affair? Have you identified and addressed your own contributions to vulnerabilities in this relationship? Consider what you're willing to give, and what you'll give up, to help this relationship succeed. Can you commit to making this relationship work in the long term even if your injured partner is struggling with this in the short term? If deep shame or excessive guilt is interfering with your ability to restore an intimate and joyful relationship with your partner, are you prepared to do whatever it takes to move past those feelings?

Additional Considerations

Concerns about the potential impact on children influence many persons' decisions about whether to stay together. What that impact might be is difficult to predict. Professionals disagree enormously about the effects of parental conflict and separation or divorce on children. One thing that is clear, however, is that many different factors come into play, from the quality of the parents' relationship and parent–child interactions before separation or divorce to the children's ages, their involvement with their parents and the parents' interactions with each other after ending the parental relationship, and how an end to the parents' relationship affects the children's economic and social well-being. It's also clear that staying together "for the sake of the children" rarely serves them well if their parents continue to have frequent and intense arguments. *Both research and clinical findings confirm that children's overall emotional well-being is best served when their parents:*

- Reduce the frequency and intensity of arguments in the home, particularly those witnessed by their children, or collaborate to minimize continuing conflicts following separation or divorce.

- Commit to not pulling their children into their conflicts and disagreements while together, or during or after separation and divorce.

Whether you decide to move forward together or separately, commit to moving on in a healthy way for the sake of your children as well as for yourselves.

For some people, the decision about whether to stay in a relationship is also strongly influenced by personal or religious values. If you're struggling with such issues, it can be helpful to talk with carefully selected friends, family members, or professional counselors or to seek spiritual direction from a trusted spiritual adviser. But be careful about placing *too much* weight on any advice you receive, no matter how well intended. Ultimately, you need to take responsibility for reaching and implementing your own decision.

Talk with your partner about factors you're considering as you work toward a decision and invite your partner's own evaluations. Begin by reviewing positive reasons for staying in the relationship and then identify remaining concerns and describe their importance. What would it take from each of you to address them? Finally, remember that ultimately it will require work from both of you to make your relationship succeed. Either one of you can end the relationship regardless of the other one's wishes or efforts. Similarly, either of you can undermine or sabotage the relationship by letting your partner do all the work of changing.

What If I Decide to Stay?

If you've been working through this book largely on your own, now is a good time to invite your partner again to read through the book and work with you. You may not both need to complete all the exercises at this time. But even if you've already worked through them by yourself, ask your partner to join you in identifying what put your relationship at risk and addressing these factors as fully as possible. Beyond that, if you and your partner decide to move forward together, your challenge will be to continue the efforts you began as you worked through the earlier chapters— healing the past, strengthening the present, and enriching the future. The kinds of work required have already been introduced, but certain aspects of this work, described below, will require continued effort.

Healing the Past

You began work aimed at healing the past when you and your partner first had discussions about what happened and how it impacted you both. Couples take additional steps toward healing when the involved partner accepts responsibility, expresses genuine remorse, and demonstrates efforts toward reform and when the injured partner acknowledges these. Further healing can occur as couples work through a process of release and reconciliation described in the previous chapter.

Healing from an affair requires you to develop the best understanding possible of how the affair came about. However, there comes a point at which further cycling through questions of "Why did you do it?" provides no new information, can be emotionally exhausting, and may interfere with reestablishing closeness and moving on together. Does the information you have about why the affair occurred give you and your partner guidance about what you each need to do differently? If so, it may be time to let go of further questions about why the affair occurred to focus instead on rebuilding the future.

Finally, it's important to remember that healing from the past is a process that will likely continue even after you've worked through issues of forgiveness or letting go and reached a clear decision to move forward together. There will likely be times in the future when you or your partner remember the affair and its impact with feelings of deep hurt, sadness, or guilt. At those times, try to focus on how far you've already come in the healing process, regain your vision of where you and your partner want to be in the future, and recommit to doing what it takes in the moment to tolerate or work beyond those feelings.

Strengthening the Present

In previous chapters, you considered what it would take to reduce the risk factors and increase the protective factors in you, your partner, and your relationship. Review your responses to the exercises in those chapters and examine how you've addressed aspects of yourselves that contributed to your relationship becoming vulnerable to an affair. Have you strengthened aspects of yourselves that are essential to recovery? Strengthening the present doesn't mean trying to get back to where you were; it means making the most of where you are. It involves more than reducing conflict and requires creating opportunities for intimacy and joy. It requires implementing everything you've learned about maintaining a secure and loving relationship and continuing in those efforts, especially when it's difficult and you may least feel like doing so.

Enriching the Future

Couples can stay together but remain stuck. Moving forward requires a vision of where you want to be and a road map for getting there. On one level, the road map may involve specific plans for dealing with setbacks and getting back on track. On another level, moving forward involves envisioning the bigger picture of your long-term future together. You and your partner will feel more emotionally connected when you share a vision of how you want to develop as a couple or family. Talk with your partner about your dreams of how you'd like to move forward and what you're willing to do to make your dreams a reality.

How Do I Regain Trust?

Trust can be one of the last important qualities to return to a committed relationship after an affair. Some people struggle with this more than others because they were wounded or betrayed in previous relationships. Some people struggle more with earning or maintaining trust because of tendencies to be secretive or to test the boundaries of relationship rules or expectations. By and large, most couples enter committed relationships with high levels of mutual trust. However, once an affair has occurred, trust can be extraordinarily difficult to recover. Rebuilding trust takes time, and progress along the way often requires small, incremental steps such as those listed in the box on the next page.

It's helpful to distinguish among different levels or kinds of trust. Apart from issues of fidelity, you or your partner may have concerns about trust regarding specific issues or areas in your relationship. For example,

Efforts to regain trust include the following:

- As the injured partner:

  o Taking small gradual risks and tolerating initial discomfort

  o Resisting urges to "check on" your partner behind their back (for example, not looking through the involved partner's phone without their permission)

- As the involved partner:

  o Eliminating secrecy

  o Honoring relationship boundaries

  o Keeping agreements with your partner about specific issues in your relationship

can you trust your partner to listen when you're discussing an issue? Can you trust your partner to treat you with courtesy and respect when you're around others? Can your partner be trusted to honor agreements you've made to address factors that put your relationship at risk? If you tell your partner you'll be home at a given time, can your partner count on you to show up then or to call ahead of time? One way to work toward rebuilding trust is to cooperate in reaching and keeping agreements on specific issues or in particular areas one at a time. As trust grows in specific areas, this often creates a sense of hope and begins to rebuild feelings of trust on a more general level as well.

Rebuilding Trust When You're the Injured Partner

Trust involves moving forward in the face of uncertainty. You need to decide whether you're willing to work toward rebuilding a relationship of mutual trust. Doing so inevitably involves accepting some degree of risk of being hurt again—no matter how small. Rebuilding trust doesn't require no longer worrying; instead, it involves identifying gradual risks you're willing to take and your ability to tolerate the discomfort of never knowing for certain that you couldn't be betrayed again. Think about the different situations that contribute to your feeling mistrustful of your partner's pledge to remain faithful. List these situations in order of difficulty—from those that trigger only low levels of apprehension to those that trigger the highest. When are the times you feel least secure? Which risk factors do you feel least confident about having eliminated? Talk with your partner about your fears and discuss additional steps either of you could take to reduce those risks.

What are the smallest steps you're willing to take now toward reestablishing trust? Consider working toward specific agreements with your partner around issues separate from fidelity. For example, would it help to rebuild trust if your partner kept agreements about spending time with you or the children instead of at work or with others? Would your relationship feel more secure if your partner talked with you about hurt feelings or decisions you're both facing in your relationship? Following through on such commitments may not eliminate your trust issues around fidelity— but these efforts can provide an initial foundation for rebuilding trust on a more general level.

Separate from your partner's efforts, what will you have to do on your own to tolerate discomfort in accepting some risk, no matter how small? For example, would it help to remind yourself of your partner's efforts when you're struggling with feelings of mistrust? What would be some indicators along the way that you were making progress in rebuilding trust? While trying to rebuild trust, recognize that this will take time. Look for opportunities to move forward in small increments. If you continue to have difficulty in working toward a trusting relationship, review the discussion in Chapter 11 regarding barriers to moving on and strategies for getting unstuck.

Rebuilding trust is a process that evolves over time. After first learning of your partner's affair, any level of uncertainty about your partner's future behaviors may feel overwhelming. That's why initially it's important that your partner go "above and beyond" in working to regain your trust by being completely open with you about what they're doing, who they're with, where they're going, and so on. However, as you learn more about your partner over time and hopefully observe evidence of their commitment to earning back your trust, you'll gradually need to reduce the amount of detail you pursue about your partner on a daily basis. It's unlikely you'd find your relationship to be satisfying or joyful if you felt compelled in the long-term to check up on your partner multiple times each day. And over time, your partner would likely resent feeling monitored, controlled, and mistrusted no matter how much they've worked toward change. So the process of restoring trust changes over time as your partner reliably demonstrates trustworthy behavior and you take small, informed steps of your own to accept some degree of uncertainty.

Regaining Your Partner's Trust after You've Had an Affair

Taking responsibility for the affair and promising to change are necessary but usually not enough to regain your partner's trust. Being faithful now doesn't prove that you won't be unfaithful down the road. To regain your partner's trust, you have to commit to reform in the ways described in Chapter 11 and then take steps to go beyond these essential commitments. For example, it's not enough to eliminate secrets; you need to work at being completely open, particularly in terms of your interactions with the outside affair partner or anyone else your partner may regard as a potential threat. Not only is it important not to engage in emotional or physical intimacy with anyone other than your partner, or beyond the boundaries the two of you have set if you've agreed to a nonmonogamous relationship; you need to adhere to tighter boundaries that show that you won't even get close to having a special relationship with someone else. Remember that your partner may no longer be willing or able to accept some of your behaviors that were okay in the past—for example, spending time away from home by yourself or with friends—because those behaviors serve as reminders of a whole range of risk factors that may have contributed to your affair.

You may have found it easier to accept restrictions or tolerate your partner's mistrust earlier, when your partner first learned of your affair, but now find it increasingly difficult to deal with your partner's continuing mistrust. Talk with your partner about the times they struggle with mistrust. Explore ways in which you can begin rebuilding trust by identifying specific concerns your partner has and then reaching agreements together about specific behaviors you're able and willing to perform. Remember that your partner's ability to trust you will probably develop more slowly than you want.

Darius's affair occurred after several months of Jada's spending most weeks on the opposite coast helping her mother recover from heart surgery. On one occasion when Jada had been gone for several weeks, he accepted a colleague's invitation for dinner at her home and they subsequently spent the night together. Darius confessed the incident to Jada several weeks after she returned. In the difficult months that followed, they identified numerous factors that had made their relationship vulnerable to an affair. Both partners wanted to salvage their relationship if possible, and they rapidly moved to place limits on outside intrusions and set aside time for themselves.

Regaining trust required special efforts by both partners. Darius recognized that, given both Jada's long-standing concerns about his behaviors with women and his affair, he needed to be completely open with Jada about interactions with others even if this sometimes caused her to feel more distressed. He went to considerable lengths to keep her informed of where he was during the day, whether he needed to work late, and—if so—who else would be there with him. Over time, Jada became more comfortable with less information while Darius still kept himself accountable. Jada also worked to understand her own fears better and to identify reasons for feeling more confident in herself. Her next visit to her mother renewed her discomfort and presented the couple with difficult challenges, but also opportunities to identify better ways of staying connected during Jada's absences and communicating about their needs for each other. Within a year after Darius's affair, they had restored their relationship and, by addressing previous risk factors, had created a healthier and more resilient relationship together.

What If I Decide to Leave?

If either one of you decides to end your relationship, how you implement that decision will influence not only how constructive or damaging the process is, but potentially also how well you move forward after the separation or divorce is complete.

Moving on separately in a healthy way requires two things from you and your partner:

1. Anticipating practical and emotional issues for you and others directly affected by this decision
2. Maintaining your dignity by treating each other with courtesy and civility

The latter may seem undeserved by your partner and may require extraordinary effort on your part, but the long-term benefits of maintaining your self-respect by behaving civilly during this difficult process are well worth the struggle, particularly if you have children together.

What Will I Need to Plan For?

The list of items to consider when ending a long-term relationship is potentially endless, but broad themes include pragmatic concerns related to living arrangements, finances, division of property, and informing others. Special themes that we'll consider separately include how to care for your children and how to care for yourself.

If possible, you and your partner should discuss where each of you will live in the short term during the separation process and in the longer term once the separation or divorce is complete. Determine who will be responsible for which bills until the end of your relationship is finalized—including house or car payments, credit card debts, clothing or medical expenses for the children, and so on. Initial discussions about shared property may be useful, particularly as these relate to major purchases you might face when setting up separate households. Avoid arguing over "pots and pans"—relatively small items of little emotional value that can easily be replaced. If you and your partner have managed to maintain a cooperative relationship, you may be able to work toward moving on separately largely on your own or with the help of a mediator. If you're struggling to work together constructively toward ending your relationship, consider getting help from a professional counselor.

At some point you'll need to inform others of your decision to end your relationship. Work through that process slowly, beginning with those who most need to know (for example, members of your family or possibly your employer). Avoid going into detail about the struggles you and your partner have had. Talking about your partner in negative ways can place friends or even family members in a difficult position, and down the road you and your partner may want to interact together with these people at large family events like graduations, weddings, or funerals.

How Should We Care for Our Children?

The most important principle in caring for your children is this: *Place your children's well-being above your own hurt and anger.* Help them maintain caring and loving relationships with both parents. Try to minimize the disruption in your children's lives and help them anticipate what changes are inevitable and how you intend to help them adjust to these changes. Consider letting neighbors or the parents of your children's best friends know about your decision because they may be able to provide your children some relief or stability when things are particularly chaotic for you and your partner. You may also want to inform your children's teachers, particularly if a child has experienced a recent increase in school-related problems.

Children often feel powerless and vulnerable when their parents separate or end their relationship. They worry about where they'll live, where they'll go to school, whether they'll have to give up their friends and make new ones, how often they'll get to see each parent, and so on. Younger children are particularly vulnerable to fears of being abandoned. Children of any age are susceptible to feeling responsible for their parents' decision to separate or divorce. They're also likely to feel angry—either because of the negative impact on their own lives or, especially among older children, from a moral perspective—and wish that somehow their parents had "done better." It's not uncommon to see signs of anxiety (for example, tearfulness or difficulties with sleeping), anger (for example, temper tantrums and verbal or physical aggression toward others), withdrawal or clinginess, or rebellion against parental rules. It's also not uncommon for anger to be expressed more openly toward the custodial parent, in part because that relationship may be seen by the child as safer and more secure.

Offer your children an opportunity to talk about their feelings and listen without judgment. Offer encouragement and reassurance that, with time and effort, things will improve and become more stable. Most of all, remember that a critical factor in your children's adjustment will be how well you and your former partner collaborate in taking care of and making decisions about your children. Avoid putting your child in the middle of any conflicts between you and your partner as a go-between or mediator. And be sure not to use them as a resource for venting your frustrations or make them choose between your partner and you.

How Should I Care for Myself?

In many ways, the emotional effects of separation or divorce for adult partners are similar to those for their children. You may feel powerless and vulnerable and may worry about where you'll live, how much money you'll have, how often you'll see your children, whether your family or friends will desert you, and whether you'll find a new partner. You may feel abandoned or rejected by your partner. You may feel profoundly guilty for ending your relationship or causing your partner to end it. Anxiety and depression may result in difficulties in sleeping, concentrating at work, or taking care of yourself such as by sticking to good nutrition and exercise.

Preparing ahead of time by working through the logistics and strengthening social and emotional support from friends and family can keep these negative reactions from becoming too severe or too long-lasting. Time may not heal all wounds, but it helps. Review the important aspects of self-care described in Chapter 5. In what ways are you not caring for yourself? Try to anticipate how you could offset losses of various relationships by cultivating others. Try to remember that, beyond initial grieving, ending a close relationship can provide opportunity for growth and renewal elsewhere.

> Callie and Jared struggled for a year to make sense of Jared's affair with a young tenant in a duplex he had owned since he was single. Both partners wanted to save their relationship, if possible, and agreed to counseling together. Callie and Jared shed many tears in the early sessions— Callie from her deep hurt and Jared from his equally deep remorse. In exploring the context for Jared's affair, they both gained insight into Jared's lifelong pattern of seeking out situations that provided excitement while risking his own welfare. By engaging in his affair, Jared had risked not only his own well-being, but Callie's too.
>
> Jared developed a better understanding of his pattern of risky

behaviors and took important steps to set boundaries for himself. He continued to work faithfully at supporting Callie and regaining her trust. Callie didn't want their relationship to end, but Jared's lifelong impulsivity reflected an enduring risk she couldn't tolerate. After months of challenging her own feelings, Callie concluded that although she would always care for Jared and regard him as a friend, she could never regain the depth of intimacy or admiration for him that she viewed as essential. She wanted a partner who prized her and aspired to the same vision of a committed relationship she had—not someone who would labor to accommodate it. Following several more months of struggling over what to do, they tearfully decided to end their relationship and move on separately. Although their decision was initially painful, both partners agreed that they were able to move on in a healthier way because of the work they had done to understand themselves and each other better.

What If I Still Can't Make Up My Mind?

After carefully evaluating all of these factors related to moving forward, you may still have difficulty making a decision. *Common situations leading to continued difficulties in making a decision include the following:*

- Your partner has undertaken important changes, but there are still too many unresolved issues for you to feel confident that your relationship can work in the long run.

- Your partner continues to behave in ways that interfere with restoring trust or intimacy, but these haven't yet convinced you that the only remaining course is to move on separately.

- Your partner has done everything you've asked and you've let go of your deep hurt and anger, but you haven't recovered feelings of intimacy and aren't sure they'll ever come back.

- Your relationship isn't so bad that you can't tolerate it, and you're reluctant to end it because of the negative impact you believe this would have on your children.

Resolving the first two problems may require obtaining additional information and engaging your partner in the process. For example, if important issues remain unresolved, talk with your partner about your lingering concerns and explore what you could each do to resolve them. If your partner is still putting your relationship at risk, confront your partner with the behaviors that are blocking recovery from the affair and be clear about what steps would be required for you to stay in the relationship. In both cases, consider a time line for achieving further progress and reevaluating the situation to determine whether you can reach a clearer decision about how to move forward.

If your partner is already doing everything you've asked to restore a close relationship but you remain stuck emotionally, your efforts may need to focus more on you and your own barriers to moving on. In these situations, we typically recommend continuing to work toward restoring a caring relationship to see whether feelings of intimacy return. The trauma of an affair often produces a kind of emotional numbness, and people vary in how long they take to recover their feelings. That said, there are two cautions: First, it's important to develop a reasonable time line for your feelings to return. Even with consistent effort, it may take months or even years for feelings of emotional closeness to return; no one can tell you how long is long enough to see if those feelings come back. And second, time alone will not be enough. Simply waiting for intimate feelings to return on their own, without actively working toward promoting emotional and physical closeness, is likely to fail.

Finally, if you're stuck because of concern over the potential effects on your children, consider talking to trusted friends who have ended their previous relationship and have children of ages similar to yours. Reading reputable books written from a variety of perspectives may also give you a balanced understanding of children's vulnerability and resilience to their parents' separation or divorce. (See the Additional Resources section at the end of this book regarding issues related to divorce.)

It's important not to rush into decisions or act on initial impulses before you're confident that you've considered all the relevant factors to a reasonable degree. It's also important to consider which actions are sustainable or reversible. For example, deciding to stay in your relationship for three months to collect more information may be less disruptive than separating temporarily to evaluate what that's like. It's also important, however, not to delay your decision indefinitely. Maintaining the status quo by avoiding a decision rarely makes the current situation better.

Work through the following exercises, which might help you reach an explicit decision about how to move forward and then examine how to implement your decision. In the final chapter, we'll help you step back and gain perspective on all you've worked toward and learned since the affair, as well as what to anticipate in the coming months.

EXERCISES

EXERCISE 12.1 Reaching a Decision about How to Move Forward

If you haven't yet decided what to do, this exercise may help you reach that decision. If you've already decided how to move forward, this exercise will help clarify the factors that went into your decision.

Make two lists—one recording reasons to move on together and the other including reasons to move on separately. Consider factors you identified previously in working through the exercises for Chapters 6–9. Not all factors are likely to be equally important, so it can also be helpful to assign numbers or weights to each of the items on your list—for example, 3 for very important, 2 for somewhat important, and 1 for least important. For instance, an important reason for staying together in your relationship might be:

> "My partner has shown deep remorse for the affair, and I can see the changes he's making. If he continues to work at change, I want to work hard as well at making our relationship succeed."

Alternatively, you might decide that an important reason to move on separately is:

> "Although we've generally gotten along well for most of our relationship, I think in large part we were staying together out of a fear of being alone. I want to and believe I could develop a much more loving and fulfilling relationship with someone else."

Once you've completed your lists and rated the importance of these different factors, pull this information together and see where it leads you. This decision isn't a simple mathematical process; nor is it just a matter of reason or logic. The best decisions are those that combine your reasoning along with your feelings. Be sure you give yourself time to work through this process and revisit your notes at times when you're feeling different levels of distress or optimism. That way, you're more likely to arrive at a balanced view that considers all the relevant factors and emphasizes those that you've determined to be most important.

If you and your partner are both reading this book, complete this exercise independently and then talk about where you both are in your decision. If you're leaning in different directions, this will likely lead to very difficult conversations. Take your time to think through these critical issues before initiating the discussion, but be sure to talk with your partner before reaching a final decision.

If you're reading this book alone, complete the exercise and try to get your partner to do the same. Even without reading the book or working through previous exercises, your partner may be able to list some pros and cons of staying in the relationship versus ending it. If your partner won't participate in this exercise at any level, do it alone and talk with your partner about the decision you're contemplating.

EXERCISE 12.2   Implementing Your Decision to Stay or Go

If Moving Forward Together

If you've decided to move forward together in your relationship, make a list of the things you still need to address to give your relationship the best chance of succeeding in the future. Focus on changes that each of you would need to make as individuals, changes for your relationship, and changes in relating to others around you. After listing important changes in these areas, talk with each other about specific strategies for implementing these changes. Then review your list and the steps you've each taken a month from now and then again six months later.

If Moving Forward Separately

If you've decided to move forward by ending your relationship, you'll want to do so in the healthiest way possible and will need to address both emotional and practical issues. *Your feelings will evolve over time, so agree to have several conversations with your partner about the feelings you're both having and how they change.* It's often necessary to address some of the emotional issues before moving on to pragmatic issues. Don't just focus on your hurtful or angry feelings. We've worked with couples who, while ending their relationship, talked with each other about the good things they had experienced together—for example, how they grew or what they'll miss. Those couples moved on better than others who ended their relationship in anger.

Make a list of the important practical issues you'll need to address. Some major practical issues include concerns related to living arrangements, finances, division of property, and informing others. Other important issues may include how to care for your children and how to care for yourself. It may be difficult at times for you and your partner to have constructive conversations about these critical issues, so discuss ahead of time how to make this process productive and respectful—for example, discussing these issues only on weekends, when you're both feeling rested; or addressing only one issue during a conversation so emotions don't build. Treating each other with dignity and fairness will leave each of you feeling better about the other and yourself.

13

What Lies Ahead?

Grace had been trying to listen to her friend Addie, but her mind kept wandering. "I'm totally lost," Addie despaired. "It's a nightmare, and I wish I could just wake up and find it all gone." A few weeks earlier Addie had discovered that her husband, Grant, had been having an affair for six months. Addie and Grant were now living in separate rooms of their house. "I just don't know what to do," Grace heard Addie continue. "Grant doesn't seem to be able to make up his mind. I don't think he's sleeping with her anymore, but I know they talk almost every day. I don't want to lose Grant, but I can't imagine ever getting over this. We had dreams together—everything to live for, everything to lose. How could he have done this?"

Grace debated how much to share with her friend. She and Jesse had been through a similar crisis two years earlier, following Grace's own affair. Addie didn't know about Grace's affair—but Grace certainly knew about the trauma that Addie was experiencing. Grace recalled how close she and Jesse had come to ending their relationship and how hard they had each struggled to hold on and rebuild it from scratch. It had taken three months before their shouting matches finally ended, and another six months before they had any real understanding of what had happened and why. Now, two years later, there were still heartaches when either of them remembered Grace's affair. But they were stronger and wiser now. They had renewed their commitment to each other and understood better than ever what that required of them.

Grace knew that Addie and her husband would need more help than she or Jesse could provide. But at least she could offer some *understanding of Addie's feelings and encouragement about their potential to recover. "It's a long and difficult process," Grace said softly. "But I think I can tell you about what it might look like . . . "*

What lies ahead, and how can you prepare for it? Like Grace and her husband, Jesse, you may still struggle at times with painful memories of the affair. We hope that you've also gained strength and wisdom from working through the previous chapters and have a clearer vision of how you want to move forward—either separately or with your partner. In this final chapter, we'll help you anticipate what still lies ahead. For most people, recovery from an affair continues even after they've reached decisions about how to move on. Whether with or without your current partner, knowing what challenges may arise and having some strategies for managing them can help with continuing the recovery process.

Safeguarding your current or future relationship and moving forward in a healthy way requires that you do the following:

- Anticipate setbacks involving hurt feelings and painful memories.
- Use your memories of the previous affair to prevent any recurrences.
- Avoid situations and people who place your relationship at risk.
- Use the communication skills you've gained to:
  o Express your feelings more constructively.
  o Manage conflict and reach decisions together more effectively.
- Promote physical closeness.
- Cherish your relationship.
- Stay focused on your vision for the future.
- Seek out additional help you may need for yourself or your relationship.

Anticipate Setbacks

Either you or your partner may continue to experience hurtful feelings or memories related to the affair. We hope that with time and effort these will become increasingly less frequent, less intense, and briefer in terms of their hurtful impact. Injured partners tend to struggle with hurtful memories longer than involved partners (although the opposite sometimes occurs). Some circumstances—for example, anniversaries of events related to the affair or special occasions in your own relationship—may stir up memories of the affair that have been quiet for weeks or months. Hurtful recollections of the affair don't necessarily indicate "going backward" or "starting all over again." Instead, they're more often a painful but natural part of the process of moving forward.

Anticipating setbacks and placing them in perspective can help prevent them from becoming traumatic occasions in themselves. You can use the skills you developed in Chapter 2 for dealing with flashbacks. For example, if you're the one struggling with hurtful memories, you can decide to cope with these on your own using self-care techniques, or you can share your struggles with your partner and request separate time for yourself or special time together as a way of experiencing closeness and reassurance. If you recognize that your partner is struggling with memories from the affair, you can offer acceptance of your partner's feelings, ask your partner what you could do right then that would be most helpful, reaffirm the progress you've already achieved as a couple, and reassure your partner that you'll continue to be there to move forward together as best you both can.

Make Good Use of Your Memories

Use your memories of the affair as a way of "keeping watch" or remaining vigilant—not in a fearful way, but in a healthy, protective way. Once an affair occurs, the illusion that many couples have that "it could never happen to us" has been shattered. Moving forward in a constructive way requires continuing to use what you've learned from the affair to keep you and your relationship safe. For example, if your relationship became vulnerable because you or your partner was devoting too much time to work or to others, or you drifted apart emotionally or physically at home, have you begun to slip back into an unhealthy pattern? It's important not to stray from important changes or renewed commitments that the affair may have brought about.

You can also use your memories of the affair constructively if you've decided to move on separately from your partner. For example, you may have a better understanding of what's most important to you in considering a new relationship. You may understand yourself at a deeper level and know better how to build and maintain a relationship that is less vulnerable to an affair. You may also be better prepared to recognize outside risks and know how to address them.

Viewed from this perspective, memories of the affair can be something other than just hurtful or disruptive. They can serve as a useful reminder of how to move forward in a more thoughtful and purposeful way, keeping your values and priorities in clear order.

Avoid Unnecessary Risks

No one else has as much at stake in your relationship as you do. No one else will work as hard to protect your relationship as you must. Employers and community organizations may place demands on your time. Children have endless need of your time and emotional energy. Friends may ask you to socialize separately with them. Outsiders may minimize the importance of relationship or family commitments you already have. *The world is full of potential risks and threats to your relationship.* Give your time and energy to activities and friends who support and strengthen your relationship and avoid unnecessary involvement with those who don't.

You need to take charge in actively avoiding situations that, either directly or indirectly, place your relationship at increased vulnerability to an affair. Outsiders don't need to explicitly encourage infidelity to place your relationship at increased risk; all it takes is interacting with others in ways that don't honor your relationship as your first priority. It's up to you to resist these outside influences as they arise.

Keep Communicating

Talk often and well. Common factors contributing to an affair involve emotional distance that sets in when partners start to lead parallel but disengaged lives or when resentments accumulate from ineffective strategies for dealing with conflict or reaching decisions together. Recovery from an affair forces partners to talk with each other. However, too often after the initial turmoil has subsided, couples slip back into previous communication patterns that interfered with collaboration and emotional closeness.

There are two ways of maintaining effective communication. One involves daily "connection talks" of 10 to 15 minutes as a way of learning about what's going on in each other's lives. Resist the temptation to reduce your exchanges to "How was your day?" followed by "Fine" or a similarly brief reply. Use open-ended prompts such as "Tell me about your day. What was the best part? What was the most frustrating part?" Create a time to have this discussion when you can actually listen to each other. If you wait for talk time to appear on its own, it probably won't. You have to make the time and effort to stay connected.

An additional way of maintaining effective communication is to set aside one 20- to 30-minute time each week when you check in with each other regarding relationship issues. The goal of this exchange is to ensure that each of you recognizes and addresses any issues that have developed during the week or need further discussion. This exchange can begin with the simple question "How are we doing?" This permits you to talk about things you've done well and ways in which you've felt close, as well as identifying any concerns you have. If the relationship has been going well, discuss why or how that's so. What did you most appreciate this past week? When did you feel closest? You can also use this time to discuss what's coming up in the days or week ahead that will require your working together.

Keep Touching

Work at staying physically connected. Use hugs or gentle touches throughout the day to show affection toward one another—when you first wake up, when you pass one another or work side by side, and before you go to sleep. Hold hands when sitting together on the couch or going for walks. Snuggle often. Physical closeness between partners can help to ease tensions or minor irritations that can arise from within or outside the relationship.

Make time for sexual intimacy or other forms of physical closeness. If you or your partner struggles with one or more sexual difficulties and want to work on your physical relationship, consider seeking professional help. Talk with each other about ways to maintain or revitalize your physical or sexual relationship. Remember that it's not necessary or realistic to experience "great sex" every time you and your partner are intimate. What's important is that you stay physically connected in ways that feel rewarding, pleasurable, and mutually caring.

Cherish Your Relationship

Cherishing your relationship goes beyond protecting against risks and maintaining good communication. It involves bringing a level of energy and commitment to your relationship that nurtures and strengthens your bond. Look for opportunities to be together in new and exciting ways. Think of each other during the day and find ways of expressing this to your partner—for example, with a brief text or a caring note left for your partner to discover during the day. Think back to the best times of your relationship, when you felt most special—perhaps to your initial courtship or times later in the relationship when you felt a special connection between the two of you. What did you each say and do that let the other one feel cherished? Cherishing each other requires resisting the temptation to take each other for granted. It requires some imagination and creativity, supported by enduring commitment.

Stay Focused on Your Vision

There are two kinds of thinking that get couples into trouble. The first involves adopting a wait-and-see attitude. Individuals adopting this attitude create an uncertainty in themselves and in their partners. Waiting for something bad to happen gets in the way of making good things happen. Eventually, in most relationships, bad things *do* happen at one level or another. They're more likely to happen if there's a void in the relationship because one or both partners are holding back to see what develops before committing to a vision for the future; moreover, the impact of negative events is greater because there isn't a strong foundation of continued positive interactions to help offset or cushion them.

The second kind of thinking that gets couples into trouble is the throwing-in-the-towel attitude during times of conflict. Following an affair, some couples restore a fragile alliance but don't do the daily work to make things solid between them. Their relationship remains vulnerable to the smallest stressor, minor disagreements rapidly escalate into major conflicts, and either partner may threaten to end the relationship. Threats of ending the relationship have a destructive impact that lasts well beyond the situation in which they're made—even when partners later apologize and "take back" what they've said. Resist the temptation to make such threats, no matter how hurt or angry you feel in the moment. The best way to resist despair and impulses to give up is to keep a clear vision of how far you've come and where you want to go. It's okay to get blown off course, so long as you know where you're headed and can reset your direction.

Seek Out Additional Help If Needed

Recovery from an affair is rarely a smooth process. The learning of new skills and the changing of ingrained patterns essential for moving forward rarely occur all at once. You should anticipate going back and rereading chapters of this book as you move forward. Previous issues will reemerge—sometimes in their original form, sometimes in a slightly new form. New issues will emerge as well, but many of these can be addressed by using the resources that you've already developed by working through the previous chapters.

It's not necessary that you work through recovery on your own. If you and your partner have decided to move on together, it's important that you draw on each other for comfort and strength as you move forward. You may also draw on the support of your closest friends with whom you've shared information about your struggles, seeking their support of your relationship during your most difficult times. Finally, it may be helpful to seek out assistance from those with special expertise in recovering from relationship wounds—for example, a mental health counselor or other helping professional—either separately or together, to deal with the special challenges you're continuing to face in moving forward. (Consider rereading our guidance on how to do this at the end of Chapter 5, and also consider the professional organizations listed in the Additional Resources on page 281.)

Final Words

In our own experience as therapists, we've never stopped admiring the deep values and profound commitment shown by individuals and couples who have approached us for help in making good decisions following an affair. Their openness in baring their wounds and genuineness in seeking help in moving forward have been testaments to their strength. We've often been more confident in their ability to reach and implement healthy decisions about moving forward than they have, and we've rarely been disappointed.

In our final words to you, we want to voice our confidence in your ability to make the best decisions in your own life about how to move forward from this affair. We don't underestimate how difficult this struggle will be. We know that there may be times when you continue to feel hurt, angry, sad, anxious, or even hopeless. We also know that by working through the chapters and exercises we've offered here, you've already shown a level of commitment that distinguishes you from others who give up early on or rush to a "quick fix" without doing the hard work of figuring out what went wrong and then embracing a more complete and more difficult rebuilding process.

You can do this. We know this from our experience of watching countless others do what first seemed impossible. We want you to know that *you* can do this as well. You're not alone. Be patient, be persistent, and be strong. Most important, hold on to hope. You've already survived the worst. We're confident that you can now create the best.

Additional Resources

Finding a Therapist Near You

Note: General guidance for identifying a therapist for you—either as an individual or as a couple—is offered at the end of Chapter 5 in the section on finding help (pages 112–113). Below we list therapist-locator websites from various professional mental health associations. A web-based search may identify similar associations in your community. The emergence of telehealth services may also expand the network of therapists available to address your specific needs.

American Psychological Association
locator.apa.org

American Association for Marriage and Family Therapy
www.therapistlocator.net

Australian Psychological Society
www.psychology.org.au

British Psychological Society
www.bps.org.uk/find-psychologist

Books

Strengthening Your Relationship

Christensen, A., Doss, B. D., & Jacobson, N. S. (2014). *Reconcilable differences* (2nd ed.). New York: Guilford Press.
Doherty, W. J. (2013). *Take back your marriage: Sticking together in a world that pulls us apart* (2nd ed.). New York: Guilford Press.

Enright, R. D. (2019). *Forgiveness is a choice: A step-by-step process for resolving anger and restoring hope.* Washington, DC: American Psychological Association.

Gottman, J. M., & Silver, N. (2015). *The seven principles for making marriage work.* New York: Harmony Books.

Johnson, S. (2008). *Hold me tight: Conversations for a lifetime of love.* New York: Little, Brown.

Dealing with Relationship Challenges

SEXUAL INTIMACY

Gottman, J., & Gottman, J. S. (2007). *And baby makes three: The six-step plan for preserving marital intimacy and rekindling romance after baby arrives.* New York: Three Rivers Press.

Metz, M. E., & McCarthy, B. W. (2020). *Enduring desire: Your guide to lifelong intimacy.* New York: Routledge.

COUPLE FINANCES

Felton, M., & Felton, C. (2011). *Couples money: What every couple should know about money and relationships.* Scotts Valley, CA: CreateSpace.

CHILDREN AND ADOLESCENTS

Duffy, J. (2019). *Parenting the new teen in the age of anxiety.* Miami, FL: Mango Publishing.

Forehand, R. L., & Long, N. (2010). *Parenting the strong-willed child: The clinically proven five-week program for parents of two- to six-year-olds* (3rd ed.). New York: McGraw Hill.

Kazdin, A. E. (2008). *The Kazdin method for parenting the defiant child.* Boston: Houghton Mifflin Harcourt.

Dealing with Individual Challenges

EMOTIONAL HEALTH

Abramowitz, J. S. (2021). *The family guide to getting over OCD: Reclaim your life and help your loved one.* New York: Guilford Press.

Miklowitz, D. J. (2019). *The bipolar disorder survival guide: What you and your family need to know* (3rd ed.). New York: Guilford Press.

Sheffield, A. (2003). *Depression fallout: The impact of depression on couples and what you can do to preserve the bond.* New York: Quill.

Thieda, K. N. (2013). *Loving someone with anxiety: Understanding and helping your partner.* Oakland, CA: New Harbinger.

PHYSICAL HEALTH

Kivowitz, B., & Weisman, R. (2018). *Love in the time of chronic illness: How to fight the sickness and not each other.* Los Angeles: Rare Bird Books.

Issues of Diversity

Diggs, A., & Paster, V. (2000). *Staying married: A guide for African American couples.* New York: Kensington.

Dolan-Del Vecchio, K. (2008). *Making love, playing power: Men, women, and the rewards of intimate justice.* Berkeley, CA: Soft Skull Press.

Harper, H. (2009). *The conversation: How Black men and women can build loving, trusting relationships.* New York: Gotham Books.

Lovelark Press. (2022). *Growing us: An LGBTQ+ guided relationship journal.* Author.

Nogales, A. (1999). *Dr. Ana Nogales' book of love, sex, and relationships: A guide for Latino couples.* New York: Broadway Books.

Shelling, G., & Fraser-Smith, J. (2008). *In love but worlds apart: Insights, questions, and tips for the intercultural couple.* Bloomington, IN: AuthorHouse.

Wang, J. T. (2022). *Permission to come home: Reclaiming mental health as Asian Americans.* New York: Balance.

Before, during, or after Divorce

Emery, R. E. (2016). *Two homes, one childhood: A parenting plan to last a lifetime.* New York: Avery.

Hawkins, A. J., Harris, S. M., & Fackrell, T. A. (2022). *Should I try to work it out? A guidebook for individuals and couples who have been thinking about divorce* (2nd ed.). Provo, UT: Family Matters Press. Free download available at *https://extension.usu.edu/strongermarriage/divorce-prevention.*

Hetherington, E. M., & Kelly, J. (2002). *For better or for worse: Divorce reconsidered.* New York: Norton.

Papernow, P. L. (2013). *Surviving and thriving in stepfamily relationships: What works and what doesn't.* New York: Routledge.

Wallerstein, J. S., & Blakeslee, S. (2003). *What about the kids? Raising your children before, during, and after divorce.* New York: Hyperion.

Index

About the Authors

Douglas K. Snyder, PhD, is Professor of Psychological and Brain Sciences at Texas A&M University, where he served as Director of Clinical Training for 20 years. He is an award-winning researcher and practitioner and maintains a private practice in couple therapy.

Kristina Coop Gordon, PhD, is Associate Dean at the University of Tennessee, where she previously served as a College of Arts and Sciences Excellence Professor and Director of Clinical Training in the Department of Psychology. An award-winning scholar and teacher, she also has a private practice specializing in couple therapy.

Donald H. Baucom, PhD, is Distinguished Professor of Psychology and Neuroscience at the University of North Carolina at Chapel Hill. One of the originators of cognitive-behavioral couple therapy, he is an award-winning teacher and mentor and maintains a private practice in couple therapy.